a guide to

alternative
medicine

Robert Eagle

BRITISH BROADCASTING CORPORATION

This book is published in conjunction with
a BBC Radio series, *Alternative Medicine*,
consisting of six 30-minute programmes,
first broadcast on Radio 4 Long Wave and VHF
on Fridays from 26 September 1980

The series is produced by Jane Wood

*Acknowledgment is due to the following for permission to
reproduce photographs:—*
AUDIO LTD biofeedback (Michael Slatford), page 36;
BRITISH SCHOOL OF OSTEOPATHY osteopath at work,
pages 86 and 87; CAMERA PRESS healer (Les Wilson),
page 12, homoeopathic medicines (Bernard Cotte), page 60;
ROBERT EAGLE herbalists, page 79; KEYSTONE PRESS AGENCY
acupuncture, page 46; SYNDICATION INTERNATIONAL
healer & patient testing brainwave activity, page 18;
JOHN TIMBERS Robert Eagle, page 4; JOHN TOPHAM
radionics practitioner, page 26; WHO Chinese
acupuncture model (D. Henrioud), page 52

Published to accompany a series of programmes
in consultation with the BBC Continuing Education
Advisory Council

©Robert Eagle 1980
First published 1980
Published by the British Broadcasting Corporation
35 Marylebone High Street, London W1M 4AA

This book is set in 10/12pt Palatino VIP
Printed in England by Whitstable Litho Ltd
Whitstable, Kent

ISBN 0 563 16454 9

Contents

The Author

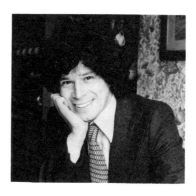

Robert Eagle is a broadcaster and journalist specialising in writing about medical matters. A graduate of Cambridge University, he regularly contributes to the *Sunday Times, World Medicine* and many other national, scientific and medical publications. As a staff writer on *General Practitioner* magazine he won the Lilly Medical Journalism Research Award in 1975. In 1979 he was awarded the Medical Journalists' Association prize for the first of several books on medical matters.

The author has written this book as a background to the BBC Radio series he presented. It contains much additional information about the therapies discussed in the programmes, and includes the views of many doctors and alternative practitioners. In the Foreword, Robert Eagle explains his own approach to the subject.

Foreword

Alternative medicine is not an easy subject to define. It is also a subject which is known by a variety of other names. While interviewing the many practitioners who contributed to the BBC Radio 4 series of programmes on which this book is based, I collected this list of alternatives to 'alternative medicine':

unorthodox medicine
unconventional medicine
traditional medicine
old wives' medicine
natural medicine
fringe medicine
complementary medicine
supplementary medicine
holistic medicine
non-scientific medicine
the new medicine
future medicine, and even
real medicine.

Several practitioners to whom I have spoken actively disapprove of the term 'alternative medicine'. They suggest that the various therapies which come under this heading are not so much alternatives to orthodox medicine as additions to it, and they are worried lest people should think that the alternative therapies can never be used with more conventional medical techniques.

Unfortunately, there is no single word which fits our subject any better than 'alternative'. For instance, can we still apply the words 'unconventional' or 'unorthodox' to a technique like acupuncture, which is now being used in several major National Health Service pain clinics? Ten years ago, acupuncture certainly was most unorthodox, but a great deal has happened since then. Therapies which were once scorned by the medical establishment as 'unscientific' are now being subjected to scientific scrutiny, and therapies which were once on the fringes of respectable medical practice appear to be moving into the mainstream.

For our purposes, alternative medicine can be taken to mean alternatives to drugs and surgery, which are the main techniques of conventional medicine. Sometimes they may prove to be real alternatives, helping when drugs or surgery have failed. But just as often they should be seen as additional therapies, extending the range of possibilities open to sick people.

Another way of describing alternative medicine would be to say that it included all the therapies which were not taught to students at medical schools. Although many contributors to our programmes were qualified doctors, some of whom work in the National Health Service, they learned their alternative therapies independently of their official medical education. However, looking ahead, it will perhaps not be long before some of the therapies we mention do enter the medical-school syllabus.

There are several reasons why the therapies which we shall be describing have not been widely recognised and practised by the medical profession, apart from the fact that doctors have never been taught them. Some therapies are claimed by their practitioners to rely on mysterious energies unknown to Western science. Traditional acupuncture, for instance, is said to work by manipulating the flow of a vital energy, called *Chi*, which flows along channels in the body quite beyond the ken of any anatomist. Healing by laying on of hands appears to rely on a healing energy which passes from healer to patient. And homoeopathy claims that some of its most powerful medicines are those which have been diluted so many times that not one molecule of the original medicinal substance is left in the remedy given to the patient. Not surprisingly, most medical scientists are unwilling to accept that such energies exist, especially as their existence would stand orthodox scientific ideas of anatomy and physiology on their heads. The manipulative therapies like osteopathy and chiropractic do not rely on unknown energies, but they have traditionally been mistrusted by doctors because many manipulators used to make wild claims that their treatment could cure just about every disease under the sun. Hypnosis has been shunned, not so much because it does not work as because it has been practised by all manner of chancers and cabaret artists: one of its pioneers, Anton Mesmer, was almost certainly a highly gifted hypnotist, but he dragged himself and his therapy into disrepute by dressing himself up in flowing robes and conducting his sessions as if they were a cross between a charade and a seance. Herbal medicine and traditional forms of medicine such as the Asian Unani-Tibb and Ayurveda are still widely practised throughout the Third World, but they have declined in popularity in the 'developed' Western world because doctors have turned to synthetic chemical compounds instead.

Most of our alternative therapies have been scorned because they appear to rely on forces like magic, superstition, religion and folklore, which just do not fit in with most contemporary scientists' idea of reality. This is a pity, because these alternative therapies very often work. Some readers may complain that by giving credence to unorthodox practices I am encouraging quacks to exploit gullible, sick people. Well, I shall be offering and quoting some advice as to how one can avoid quacks and select competent alternative practitioners. I should also like to quote one of our contributors, the medical researcher Dr David Bowsher of Liverpool University:

'I think it's rather difficult nowadays to know what to call conventional and what to call unconventional medicine. This is probably a good thing because the distinction is becoming blurred. I think that any treatment at all which claims to have any effect should be looked at dispassionately and objectively by people who know what it is doing. The only way you can test things is by looking at them. It's no use refusing to have any truck with something just because it has been done by someone who is a bit way out.'

Not a great deal of recent scientific research has been made into most of the alternative therapies, but I shall outline what has been done. And we should not forget that academic attitudes change rapidly. The author Brian Inglis told me that, when he wrote his book *Fringe Medicine* fifteen years ago, he was strongly advised to drop his chapter on acupuncture. It's Chinese, way out and just doesn't make sense, he was told. Remarkably enough, of all the therapies he described in that book, acupuncture is the one which has since attracted the most scientific attention throughout the world, with fresh papers on it appearing regularly in leading medical journals.

A few sceptical individuals whom I interviewed suggested to me that the current interest in alternative medicine was no more than a fashion, a journalistic vogue dreamed up by discontents and writers such as myself. Admittedly, it is very difficult to determine whether more people are seeking unorthodox medical treatment today than, say, twenty years ago. Because alternative medicine is largely practised outside the medical establishment, very few statistics are obtainable. Nevertheless, to judge by the number of alternative practitioners in the market, alternative medicine appears to be booming. Twenty years ago, the number of people practising acupuncture in the United Kingdom could be counted on the fingers of one hand; today, there are more than three hundred who have been through training courses, and probably many others who have taught themselves. Similarly, there are about 750 trained osteopaths, and the osteopathic organisations believe that there is at least that number again practising without any real qualifications. Membership of the various religious and lay associations which represent healers totals more than ten thousand, and although some healers may belong to more than one group, I know others who belong to no association at all. There are still many more doctors – about sixty thousand on the General Medical Council's register – than alternative practitioners, but there cannot be many towns now without a resident acupuncturist, healer, osteopath, chiropractor or herbalist. The Asian immigrant community also has its own alternative practitioners. There are about forty *hakims* in Britain practising traditional Muslim and Hindu medicine, as well as numerous unqualified Asian herbalists working informally or part time.

As the Government is currently spending around £10,000 million a year on the National Health Service, it might seem strange that people should need these alternatives. But the problems which are taken to alternative practitioners are largely those which are not successfully treated by conventional medicine. Back-ache, migraine, skin diseases, allergies, arthritis and rheumatism: these complaints make up the majority of cases that are brought to the alternative practitioner.

There is little in the way of hard statistical evidence to say that people suffering from these diseases do any better, or any worse, from an alternative therapy than from the National Health Service. I have heard scores of accounts from patients with such afflictions who got no benefit from their doctor but were cured or helped by an alternative therapy,sometimes quite dramatically. At the same time, one reads occasional press reports of people getting jaundice from an acupuncturist's dirty needles or being tricked by some quack's false pretences. Orthopaedic surgeons and rheumatologists will occasionally report anecdotes about patients with chronic spinal conditions being made worse by a manipulator; but at the same time the osteopathic organisations claim that none of their members has ever been successfully sued for malpractice by a patient.

From the patient's point of view, one of the attractive aspects of alternative medicine is that the practitioner can generally afford to spend much more time with the patient than a National Health Service general practitioner or overworked hospital doctor. The average length of an NHS GP's consultation is six minutes, whereas most alternative practitioners reckon to spend at least quarter of an hour, and sometimes up to a full hour at the first appointment. To have someone devote their undivided attention to his problems must be of great psychological value for the patient. And many practitioners, medically qualified or otherwise, admit that having to pay for treatment may also have therapeutic value: if you feel the impact of the therapy on your wallet, you have a vested interest in wanting it to work!

Another reason some patients seek alternative help is that they are afraid of drugs or have had problems with the side effects of drugs. Dr Michael Jenkins of the Royal London Homoeopathic Hospital says that many of his patients seek homoeopathic treatment because they have not been able to tolerate the drugs they were previously prescribed, this being particularly true of patients suffering from arthritis and cancer. Since the thalidomide scandal, several widely prescribed synthetic medicines have been criticised or withdrawn, due to their unpleasant or dangerous side effects. These side effects are usually noticed only when the drug has been on the market for some years. The blood pressure and heart drug practolol, for instance, was noticed to be causing irreversible eye and gut damage and skin ulcers only after it had been prescribed to tens of thousands of patients. More recently it has come to light that normal people taking normal doses of benzodiazepine tranquillisers can become addicted to their drug, and suffer terrible withdrawal symptoms if they try to give them up. During the past decade millions of prescriptions for benzodiazepines have been issued every year by doctors who believed them to be quite safe medicines. Alternative practitioners have not been slow to capitalise on this increasing fear of synthetic drugs, and much of their publicity material stresses that alternative medicine is 'natural', 'safe' and 'without side effects'. These claims are beguiling though not always strictly true. Alternative therapies do have their hazards, which I shall mention in more detail later on.

The disadvantages of drugs have also persuaded some doctors that alternatives need to be found. Dr Alec Forbes, a consultant physician working in a National Health Service hospital in Plymouth, has become an outspoken critic of the kind of medicine which he practised himself for many years. He encourages patients to use alternative therapies, and has been persuading alternative practitioners in his part of the country to set up small health centres where they can practise together. He believes that drug-based medicine has monopolised National Health Service medical practice and that we are now paying far too high a price for it – both financially and in terms of sickness:

'It is a matter of common observation that as many as twenty per cent of patients in a hospital ward at any one time are there because of the adverse effects of the drugs they have been prescribed. That is a very high price to pay for drug therapy. If the monopoly was broken and more natural therapies which are inherently safer and cheaper than orthodox medicine were allowed in, then costs would go down and the public would have a better deal. The alternative therapies would not necessarily be any more effective than orthodox medicine, but I think we could offer more help and cause less damage if we used them more freely.'

Dr Forbes's views are echoed by Dr Malcolm Carruthers of the Maudsley Hospital, London, who has been teaching non-drug therapies such as biofeedback, autogenic training and meditation:

'I think there is a crisis of confidence in the general population and in the medical profession itself. They are becoming aware that there is not "a pill for every ill", and that the disadvantages of some drug therapies outweigh their advantages. Pills may be a convenient kind of therapy, but they are often an easy way out. They do not require the patient to change any aspect of his or her life style which may be contributing to the disease. They just switch off the danger signals.'

The techniques which Dr Carruthers uses – which I shall describe in more detail later on – are relatively new to British medicine, but their efficacy and safety have been tested scientifically and by the clinical experience of many doctors. The same cannot be said of some of the alternative therapies which we shall also be describing. Some alternative practitioners have only the most rudimentary knowledge of anatomy, physiology and pathology, and the claims they make have to be viewed with caution if not scepticism. Some say that such knowledge would be quite irrelevant to them anyway because they believe that they are working on the patient's soul or etheric body rather than the physical body. And practitioners – this applies to doctors as well as to the medically unqualified – are sometimes inclined to become so enthused by their particular therapy that they overlook the fact that the mind and body have remarkable self-healing powers which can operate quite independently of the treatment which the practitioner believes to be the cause of the cure.

What I have just said may give the impression that I view alternative medicine with a sceptical, jaundiced eye. This is not the case; but it is wise to examine any curative claims, from whatever source, with caution. I believe that the individual practitioners interviewed in our programmes and whom I quote in this book are some of the most competent around. It would have been just as easy – and possibly a great deal more fun – to pack the programmes full of exposés of out-and-out charlatans. There is no shortage of quacks. But to make a great fuss about quacks at this stage would be to run the risk of casting a blight on genuine practitioners who have a lot to offer. What they do and what they believe may often strike one as bizarre, but that does not necessarily mean that they are not doing something useful.

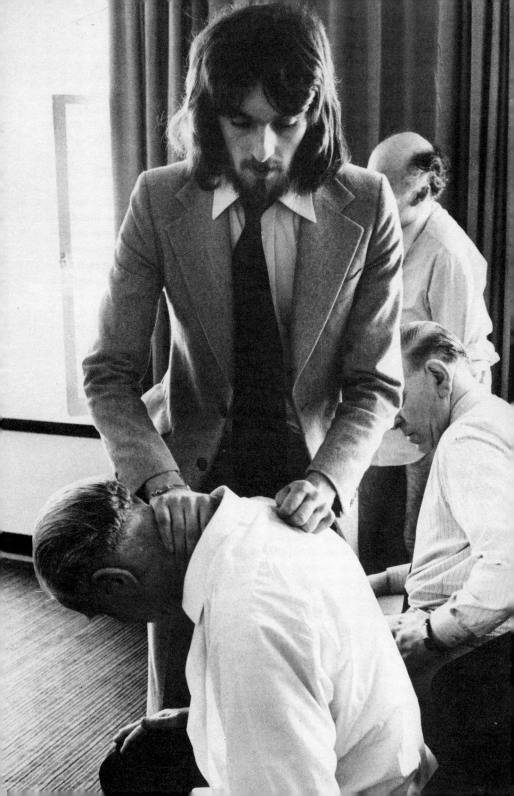

1 Healing

Let's begin by looking at one of the most remarkable alternative therapies which is also one of the simplest – healing by laying on of hands. Healing goes by several names: faith healing, spiritual healing, psychic healing, natural healing. The name which the healer chooses to use depends on where he or she believes the gift to come from. Faith healers tend to attribute it to the healer's and/or patient's religious faith; spiritual healers suggest that by healing the mind you can heal the body; psychic healers usually work by calling on discarnate spirit 'guides' and natural healers believe that there is a universal healing energy which can be tapped by almost anyone. But these titles are more confusing than helpful, and few healers fit neatly into any category. Healing techniques also vary from healer to healer, though the principal common element is that healing involves the laying on of hands.

Laying on of hands

Touching people, passing a cool hand across the fevered brow, these are natural and instinctive ways of trying to express friendship and ease pain. Indeed, many doctors have told me that they think that one of the great failings of modern, technological medicine is that doctors no longer touch their patients enough and spend too much time sitting writing prescriptions on the far side of a desk. However, although physical contact is obviously an important part of human communication, healing seems to involve something else. Patients who go to healers very often experience sensations which are much more intense than those you would expect to receive from simple hand contact. These sensations are, typically, heat, cold or

Finbarr Nolan healing a patient by laying on of hands

tingling. They may occur when the healer is touching the patient or even when his hands are at some distance from the body. Not long ago I witnessed an interesting meeting at the Centre for Pain Relief at Walton Hospital, Liverpool, which is one of the largest and most scientifically adventurous clinics of its kind in the world. The specialists there try to help patients who have failed to respond to every kind of conventional treatment, and they were interested to find out whether a healer could help some of their more difficult patients. The healer they invited was Bruce MacManaway, a well-known professional healer who lives in Scotland. Most of the patients whom MacManaway 'healed' reported sensations of heat, cold or tingling. The effect of the healer on one woman's nervous system was quite dramatic. MacManaway simply held his hand six inches above her shoulder, and this caused the palm of her hand on that arm to sweat profusely – this without any direct contact being made at all. The healer subsequently suggested that the doctors present should try laying on hands for themselves, expecting that they would be able to elicit a similar reaction. In fact, the patients felt only the normal warmth of the doctors' hands with no unusual tinglings of any kind.

This phenomenon is quite inexplicable in standard scientific terms, though it has been observed many, many times. The healers I know simply describe it as 'healing energy', and say that it is something which passes through them when they are healing.

Incidentally, several patients at that session at Walton Hospital did say that their pain went away for some time after their healing. There were no startling instant cures – but it would perhaps be unreasonable to expect startling results from a single session. No one expects a single pill to cure you for good.

A small amount of research into healing by professional scientists has been done in this country and the United States in recent years, and I shall return to this later on. But first let us hear a little bit from the healers themselves. What sort of people are they?

Those I have met are to all appearances quite normal, healthy folk, though most seem to radiate an atmosphere of ease and calm. This relaxed spirit may account for much of their success. It was certainly this characteristic of Bruce MacManaway which particularly impressed Dr David Bowsher, one of the doctors present at the healing session at Walton Hospital:

'He had the best bedside manner of anybody I have seen in some 30 years of medical experience. We all know that the sympathetic doctor is much more *effective than the unsympathetic doctor. Now if this healer had been a doctor we would have had every medical student from miles around to see him and watch his technique of bedside manner. His reassurance to patients, his making them feel at ease, the way he made them feel that they were the only person in the whole world who mattered to him, were absolutely superb.'*

MacManaway says that he discovered his healing gift in circumstances which were far from calm and relaxed. He was a young Army officer on the beach at Dunkirk and saw his men being shot up all around him. 'By some instinct,' he relates, 'I felt drawn to put my hands on them. The effects were remarkable. Somehow I was able to staunch their bleeding and ease their pain. I later found that I could detect the location of pieces of shrapnel which the field medical officers could not find. There were no X-ray facilities at hand and I found myself in great demand!'

Rose Gladden, another professional healer who works in Hertfordshire, has a rather different though no less extraordinary story of how she discovered her healing gift:

'It began when I was a child at school. I used to see angels night after night from the age of seven, magnificent angels standing in my room. Then at school, if I sat next to anyone with a pain, I would instinctively know they had a pain and feel an urge to place my hand over it. As I did so, a warmth would flow through me and the pain would disappear.

That was fifty-three years ago. I did not start doing it seriously until one day when I was nineteen. I walked into a dyers' and cleaners' shop in Edmonton, North London, to find that the owner had slumped over the counter looking very grey, very ill. I said: "What's the matter, Mr Chapman?" He said, "I have an ulcer and it's giving me terrible pain." And I thought, "Dear God, I wish I could help him." Then I heard a voice say, "You can help him. Put your hand there." I thought, "I can't do that," but the voice came again, "Go on, put your hand there." Then a little twinkling star appeared over his left shoulder and it floated down and stopped on the top of his stomach. And there it twinkled. Plucking up my courage, I said, "Mr Chapman, is that where the ulcer is?" and he said, "You're right on it." I asked him if I could put my hand there, and he said, "Of course you can." So I placed my hand over his ulcer, and as I did so I actually felt another hand go over mine and hold mine steady. My hand was filled again with a wonderful warmth. I couldn't draw it away so I just let it rest against him. Then slowly my hand was drawn to his right side and moved away, and as it did so he said, "That pain, it's gone, it's gone," and he rushed into

15

the shop next door to tell the owner. That was my first real healing and I went home walking on air.'

Rose Gladden is a remarkable person with unusual talents. She diagnoses her patients' problems by looking at their aura, a colourful halo which she says she can see around every individual. Dark areas in the aura suggest that something is amiss with the part of the body underneath, so that is usually where she begins her laying on of hands.

Another healer we interviewed was Edgar. (He asked us not to mention his full name because, unlike Bruce MacManaway and Rose Gladden, Edgar is not a professional healer. On a previous occasion when he had been interviewed by the press he had received hundreds of calls and letters from distressed people asking for help, and he had just not been able to cope with them all.) This is how he sets about examining his patients:

'It is possible to make a general diagnosis by running the hands over the head, down the neck and especially down the spine. Wherever there is an 'imbalance' I get a sensation in my hands which indicates that the problem is probably in that area of the body. If there is a trapped sciatic nerve I feel minute electric shocks. A nervous condition will make my hands prickle when they are on the patient's head. Cancer gives me a sensation of worms moving under the skin, while asthma feels like mites wriggling around. These sensations are not always very distinct, but I find that they are a useful indication of what is wrong. The patients themselves say that they get similar sensations when my hands are on them.'

Twinkling stars, auras and strange sensations may stretch your credulity. Certainly not all healers claim to experience such things. But all the healers I have mentioned so far do not fit the conventional idea of lunatic or crank. Indeed, despite their remarkable claims, they are the most down-to-earth individuals. Bruce MacManaway is a tall, portly man of military bearing with an avuncular grin. Rose Gladden is a warm, motherly person with an engaging London accent. And Edgar is a former trainer of an English hockey team, newspaper company director and management consultant. 'I'm an ordinary bloke who drinks beer,' he assured me.

I have not personally witnessed any amazing, instant cures from healing, but all the healers above have sheaves of letters and testimonials from grateful patients. Several of Edgar's regular patients are doctors and their families – he has even been asked to heal one local doctor's dog! The healers seem to be most effective at relieving pain and getting their patients to unwind and relax, though each has accounts of more dramatic and inexplicable successes. Rose Gladden, for instance, told how she had helped a young girl get rid of psoriasis, an unpleasant skin disease, after using her clairvoyant ability to unearth a forgotten but traumatic event in the girl's early life. Edgar has demonstrated his healing in front of doctors who treat patients with asthma, who found that his healing could measurably improve an asthmatic child's breathing.

Rhythms of the brain

One of the few scientists who has spent a lot of time investigating healers is Maxwell Cade of the Psychobiology Institute in London. Cade is a specialist in the design and application of instruments which measure electrical activity in the body, especially the electroencephalograph, or EEG, which records electrical activity in the brain. He has found that healers, in common with other individuals with unusual abilities, such as yogis, swamis and clairvoyants, have unusual brain-wave patterns, and that during healing these patterns somehow transfer themselves on to the persons being healed.

The electrical activity in the large cerebral hemispheres on the top of the brain varies with the state of mind. Basically, during the aroused, waking state when you are occupied with day-to-day business, it runs at about 14 to 20 cycles a second. When you close your eyes and/or relax, the rhythm falls to 7 to 13 cycles a second. Dreams or trance states usually occur when the brain appears to be ticking over slowly at 4 to 7 cycles a second, and deep sleep or unconsciousness are typified by a very slow rate of between 2 to 4 cyles a second. Each half of the brain is responsible for different human activities: the left half of the brain is more active during speech and logical, linear thinking, whereas the right side comes into play during more irrational activities such as dreaming, imagining pictures and patterns, and under hypnosis. The rapid rhythm of 14 to 20 cycles is called 'beta rhythm'; the more relaxed rate of 7 to 13 cycles is called 'alpha rhythm'; and the two even slower rates are called 'theta' and 'delta' rhythms respectively.

Generally speaking, then, when we are busying ourselves with the day's work, the left cerebral hemisphere will be most active, operating at the beta rhythm. Maxwell Cade has noticed, however, that healers regularly (and especially when they are healing) have

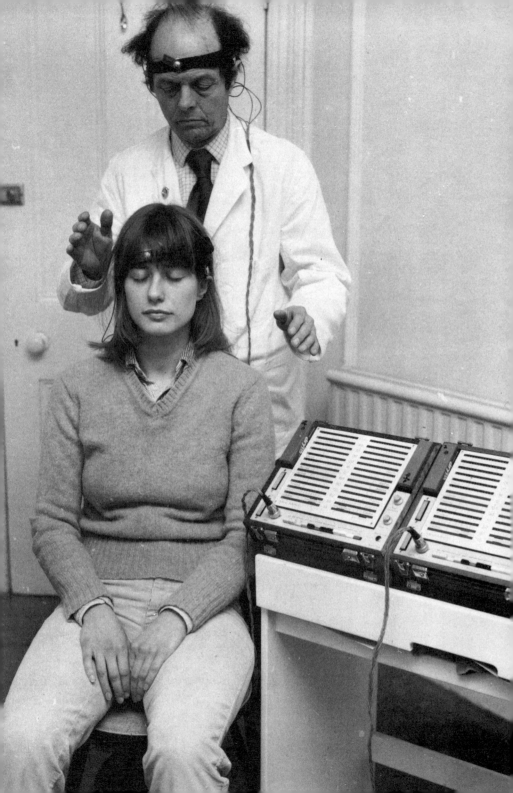

strong alpha and theta rhythms in both halves of the brain. During numerous experiments when he has wired both healer and patient up to his EEG machines, he has found that the healer's rhythms are taken up by the patient. This usually happens about ten to fifteen minutes after laying on of hands has begun, and the patient often remains in this relaxed condition for up to two or three hours.

What can healers do?

Just how or why this should happen is wide open to speculation, and Cade admits that a great deal more research should be done into this phenomenon. Is it the result of some energy moving through the healer's hands, or is it due more to the healer's personality or charisma? Whatever the cause, the result is very pleasant for the patient. Jules Cashford, volunteer patient in a public demonstration of Cade's experiments with healers, told us what she felt:

'I had been very stiff and could hardly bend forward at all at the time. Edgar [the healer] relaxed me by putting his finger on an acupuncture point on my neck and then moved his hand down my back until he found a place at the base of my spine. It was the site of an old injury, but he knew nothing about that. He said that there was "a bit of a problem here" and put his hand on it. I immediately felt a great tingling and warmth. He kept on talking, explaining what he was doing, and gradually I felt as though taken away from the place, as if it didn't matter whether I was there or whether I had this old injury in my back. I lost all fear of being ill and felt that everything was OK. As soon as Edgar had finished he told me to touch my toes. I didn't want to, but I did and there was no problem at all.'

Gifted healers obviously have a fine knack of relaxing people, and this could explain much of their success with psychosomatic complaints and with pain, a symptom which definitely tends to ebb and flow depending on the patient's state of mind. But a few other experiments with healers have shown that healing may not just be 'all in the mind'.

In 1961 Professor Bernard Grad of McGill University in Canada published a paper in the *International Journal of Parapsychology* describing how a healer had been able to make skin wounds in mice heal more rapidly than would normally be expected. The healer, a Hungarian former army officer called Oskar Estebany, was asked to place his hands over a cage of mice which had had a patch of skin,

Brainwave activity being tested in healer and patient

measuring about half an inch square, surgically removed. Two other batches of mice had been given similar wounds, but the healer was kept away from them. One of these cages was warmed very slightly to correspond with the amount of heat the 'healed' mice might have received from the healer's hands, while the third cage was left strictly alone. After two weeks the mice which had been healed had almost all lost any sign of their skin wounds, whereas lesions on the mice in the other cages had still only partially healed. So the healer appeared to have exerted an effect on his mice's health significantly beyond what might be expected from nature alone.

The same healer was later investigated by Dr Justa Smith, a biochemist working at the Human Dimensions Institute in New York. Wondering whether he could have any effect on the most basic biochemical processes she got the healer to hold flasks containing an enzyme, trypsin. She then compared the subsequent activity of the enzymes in that flask with that of similar enzymes which had been left untouched or exposed to a strong electromagnetic field. She found time and again that the healer's effect was similar to that of the electromagnetic field, even though Mr Estebany did not appear to be emanating any measurable kind of electromagnetic energy. She also got him to 'heal' flasks of enzymes which had been damaged by ultraviolet radiation, and found that after an hour in his hands the enzymes appeared to recover their previous vigour.

More recently, Dr John Kmetz of the Science Unlimited Research Foundation in San Antonio, Texas, conducted experiments with the young English psychic and healer Matthew Manning. Manning was given test-tubes containing cultures of cervical cancer cells to hold. After twenty mintues the cells lost their ability to adhere to one another. They dropped off the culture, apparently because the healer had altered the electrical charge which encourages cancer cells to stick together and create tumours. Another team of scientists at the Mind Science Foundation in San Antonio found that Manning could induce Amazonian electric fish in a tank to discharge their current, make human red blood cells resist osmosis and make gerbils run faster round the treadmills in their cages. Perhaps the most remarkable aspect of these last three experiments was that Manning did not actually handle the blood samples, animals or even their cages. He was kept in another room throughout!

These are a sample of the kind of research which has been made into healing. Of course the majority of people who go to a healer do not need to be persuaded by the results of laboratory studies. They go because they cannot find a cure elsewhere or because the healer has been recommended by friends.

Indeed, not all the scientific studies have proved successful or informative. Dr Justa Smith tried repeating her studies of Mr Estebany some months after the first series, but they could not achieve the same results. Dr Smith points out that the healer was physically not very well and had recently suffered a bereavement, factors which could have drained his powers. And Maxwell Cade and his colleagues once found that a healer whom they were testing appeared to be picking up the brain-wave patterns of the person she was healing rather than the other way round. She too was very tired at the time, perhaps in need of being healed herself. Scientists who have worked with Matthew Manning have noticed that he quickly gets bored by the rather tedious laboratory routines, and that his flagging interest may affect his results. Professor John Taylor of King's College, London, had negative results from a series of experiments he conducted with healers. He assumed that if healers emanated any kind of energy it must be electromagnetic. But he failed to find any consistent change in electromagnetic energy in the healers he studied. All this suggests that if there is a real healing energy, then it has an all too human unpredictability to it.

Healers are sometimes accused by sceptical doctors of encouraging false hopes in patients who cannot be cured. There certainly are documented cases of crippled people being so carried away by enthusiasm at a healing session that they leap from their chairs, wave their sticks in the air and cry out that they are miraculously healed. The next morning finds them as disabled as before, ruing their misplaced belief. One of the attractive aspects of laying on of hands, however, is that it does not appear to have adverse physical effects on the patient. Nevertheless, I should add a word of warning here, because healing has been known to have adverse effects on the healer. Consider this anecdote, told by one of our interviewees:

'A friend of mine discovered that he could heal and became very enthusiastic about it. All went well, until one day he met somebody who had a blinding headache and offered to help him. Well, he did succeed in clearing the person's headache completely – but he inherited it himself. He picked up the patient's headache and just could not get rid of it. This was such a nasty shock for him that he stopped healing and, as far as I know, has never taken it up since.'

The source of that anecdote is Dr Arthur Bailey, a senior lecturer in electrical engineering at Bradford University. He is also President of the British Society of Dowsers, and it was his interest in dowsing that brought him into contact with healers and an even more inexplicable form of alternative medicine – distant healing.

Medical dowsing

Dowsing is the ancient art of seeking water, metals and lost objects. It has been practised for centuries, but because it is another of those phenomena which does not appear to have a rational explanation in modern scientific terms, it is the subject of great controversy. Those who practise it claim that it is a consistently reliable way of locating objects or energies which are beyond the range of the normal five senses, but sceptics maintain that if a dowser finds anything it is by sheer luck or coincidence.

Traditionally, the dowser seeks water (or whatever else he is looking for) by walking slowly across the terrain holding a Y-shaped twig. Many dowsers today use metal divining rods or even converted metal coat hangers. When the dowser walks over an underground spring, his divining rod suddenly moves up or down, apparently of its own accord. Some healers dowse their patients by holding a pendulum over various parts of their body. Bruce MacManaway, for instance, often begins making his kind of diagnosis by holding a little pointed bob on the end of a thread held between his fingers. He dangles the bob over the vertibrae of the patient's back, and if it rotates in a clockwise direction he assumes that all is well with that vertebra, but if it swings anticlockwise he concludes that there is a trapped nerve or some other problem at that spot.

Medical dowsing is used not only by healers. Several doctors I have met – including Alec Forbes and Julian Kenyon, who were interviewed for our programmes – sometimes use a pendulum to help them decide which drug or therapy might be most useful for a particular patient. The technique can be applied either by simply thinking of the patient and dangling the pendulum over the drug, or by placing a lock of the patient's hair or some other sample such as a blood spot next to the tablets and seeing which way the pendulum swings. Generally speaking, if the pendulum rotates clockwise, then that remedy is assumed to be good for the patient, whereas if it rotates anticlockwise it is assumed not to be right. The pendulum may swing in different ways for different dowsers; for some, anticlockwise means 'yes' and clockwise means 'no'; and for others, the answer may come from the pendulum swinging to and fro rather than in a circle. But the principle remains basically the same.

Dr Bailey first became interested in the medical applications of dowsing after a homoeopathic doctor had treated him by dowsing.

'He made his diagnosis on the basis of two blood spots I sent him through the post. He would get his wife, who was better at dowsing than he was, to analyse the patient's problems with the help of a pendulum, and from that he would prescribe homoeopathic remedies, which he sent back by post. I had been very seriously ill after a bout of Asian 'flu and had not responded to conventional treatment. All I can say about his treatment is that from the day his medicine arrived, I began to improve dramatically.'

Although this personal experience convinced Dr Bailey that medical dowsing was worth looking at seriously, a single case history like this does not of course provide any real scientific proof. It would be quite reasonable to assume that his recovery occurred quite independently of the unorthodox treatment he received. Unfortunately, medical dowsers have been unwilling or unable to subject their technique to objective clinical trials to determine whether or not their success is really any better than chance. Indeed, many dowsers deliberately steer clear of investigations which might involve sceptical or hostile observers, because they find that the presence of an aggressively minded cynic can upset their ability to dowse. And although Dr Bailey is a professional scientist as well as a dowser, he admits that dowsing is 'a phenomenon without any orthodox physical explanation'.

Nevertheless, he has persisted with dowsing because it works for him. His academic colleagues at Bradford University have been sufficiently persuaded of his ability and sincerity to let him help them. He has used dowsing to locate faults in the university computer and to survey sites for the archaeological department. He also helped Post Office contractors to find underground mine shafts on a site which was to be laid with telephone cables. And in the medical field he claims to have had some useful results, too. He diagnoses people's problems with a pendulum and then tries to put them right with simple spinal manipulation:

'One woman came to me with very poor eyesight. She had been examined by orthodox medical techniques – in fact I never like to treat anyone unless they have already been screened by orthodox methods first – but although she could read large-print books, her sight was so bad that she was officially rated as blind. From my pendulum diagnosis I thought there was a pinched

nerve at the very top of her neck. I had never manipulated a neck that high up before, so I asked the pendulum what I should do. I kept my fingers very firmly crossed, and very gently eased her head and manipulated it until, according to the pendulum the trapped nerve had been freed. The whole treatment took about half an hour. The following day she told me that her eyesight had started to improve almost immediately, and within a few weeks she was reading small-print newspapers.'

This case history seemed so remarkable that I asked a doctor, John Ebbetts, former president of the British Association of Manipulative Medicine, whether he thought it could possibly be true. Rather to my surprise, he said that it was unusual but quite possible. Some patients who have suffered from whiplash injuries, in which the neck is subjected to sudden bending, do subsequently have difficulty focusing their eyes because of pressure on the nerves in the upper spinal cord which lead to the eye. Correct manipulation of the deranged joints to free the nerves can improve vision in such cases.

Distant healing

There is, therefore, one case at least where dowsing seems to have been a useful form of diagnosis. But as I have mentioned, some medical dowsers do not actually see their patients at all; they dowse at a distance over a lock of hair, blood spot or sometimes just a photograph of the patient. Dowsers looking for water may use a similar technique; rather than surveying the site itself, they begin by swinging a pendulum over a map of the site, and claim that the results are often almost as good as on-the-spot dowsing. If this is the case, then dowsing must be more than a highly attuned sensitivity to electrical currents or magnetic fields in the earth or the human body; dowsing-at-a-distance takes us into the realms of telepathy and clairvoyance. But even this vague terrain of the 'paranormal' has its practitioners and satisfied patients who believe not only that disease can be diagnosed at a distance, but also that it can be treated at a distance.

Praying for someone's health is the most ancient and best-known kind of distant healing, and it doubtless does people good to think that others far away are thinking good thoughts about them. The healers I have quoted all do distant healing as well as laying on of hands, but their technique is not the same as in conventional kinds of prayer. Edgar, for instance, keeps photographs or locks of hair from his distant patients, and during the course of the day he will hold his pendulum over this item and visualise the patient in question. When the pendulum starts to swing, he believes that he is 'in tune' with the patient, and he sets about healing them by placing his hand over the photograph or lock of hair.

Absurd, you may think. Nevertheless, I have spoken to several of his patients who firmly believe that his distant healing works, and cite instances of aches, pain and even hay fever that clear up quite suddenly after Edgar had, unknown to them, begun his distant healing. Maxwell Cade, the scientist whose studies of healers' brain-wave rhythms I mentioned earlier in this chapter, set up experiments in which Edgar at his home in the Midlands was asked to give distant healing to a group of volunteers wired up to Cade's EEG machines in London. Shortly after Edgar began his healing, thinking of each 'patient' in turn at fifteen-minute intervals, their brain rhythms in most cases changed to the kind of pattern Cade had previously seen in patients undergoing laying on of hands. In a long-term experiment currently being conducted in the United States, a group of healers are seeing if they can help people reduce their high blood pressure by distant healing. The experiment is in the charge of Dr Robert Miller, a former professor at the Georgia Institute of Technology in Atlanta. Some patients are receiving distant healing, whereas others are not, though all are being monitored regularly by their doctors. The experiment is also a 'double blind', meaning that neither the doctor nor the patients themselves are told whether they are receiving healing or not. As it is a long-term study which began only in 1979, the final results are not yet available, but preliminary results from the first few months of the study suggest that the patients receiving distant healing are reducing their blood pressure more than those who are not. In the control group – that is, the patients who are not getting distant healing – four had experienced no significant change and six had improved. In the treated group, three had experienced no significant change, and fourteen had improved. There seems to be a trend, therefore, in favour of distant healing, though it is not statistically significant. It is also interesting that more than two-thirds of the patients are improving, *whether or not they are treated*. Perhaps we can deduce from this that simply knowing that there is a fifty-fifty chance that a healer is working on you is likely to improve your blood pressure! This would be an example of the so-called placebo response, which occurs in trials of every kind of medical therapy and which I shall discuss in more detail in the next chapter.

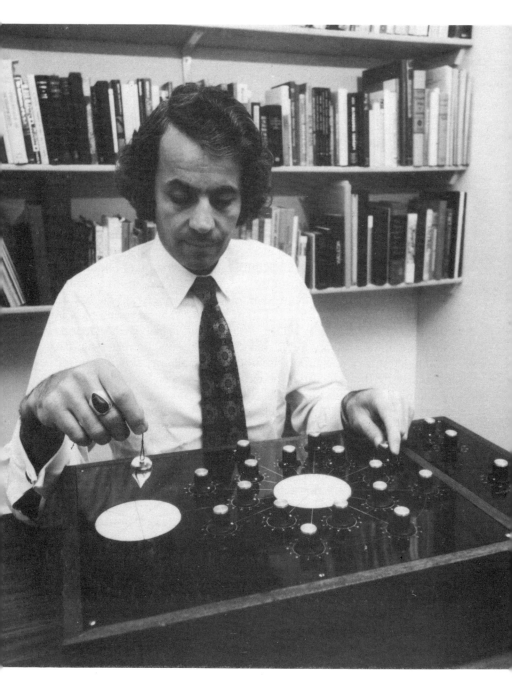

Radionics

Distant healing is combined with dowsing in one of the most esoteric alternative therapies, radionics. The founder of radionics was an American doctor, Albert Abrams, who, until he began dabbling in such strange phenomena, had enjoyed much professional respect as a physician in San Francisco. He had been professor of pathology at Stanford University and president of his city's Medico-Chirurgical Society.

To outline his work very briefly, he found that he could diagnose many illnesses simply by percussing various parts of his patient's abdomen. Percussion with a finger or rubber mallet is a standard medical technique, and the doctor can tell by the hollowness or dullness of the sound resulting from percussion the condition of the organs underneath. But Abrams developed his percussive technique to the point where he claimed he could diagnose a whole range of illnesses by percussing the abdomen, whether or not those diseases had any obvious physical connection with that part of the body. The very odd thing was that this technique only worked when his patients were facing west!

Dr Abrams wondered whether this might have something to do with the patient's orientation in the earth's electromagnetic field, and he began a series of experiments whose results convinced him that disease was indeed an electromagnetic phenomenon and that it could be cured by electromagnetic means. He found that he could diagnose particular diseases from a tissue sample wired up to a device which basically consisted of a set of variable resistors and dials. Samples of hair or blood spots were sufficient for him to diagnose the patient's complaint with this machine. These were the early days of radio, and Abrams speculated that he was able to diagnose in this way because human tissues emanated energy at a frequency similar to radio waves. He designed, and later manufactured a machine called 'the Oscilloclast', which subjected the patient to mild, high-frequency electric currents.

Dr Abrams' black box, as the machine became known, attracted a great deal of publicity, none of which helped to improve his standing with his professional colleagues, who were outright sceptics almost to a man. His ideas were taken up later not so much by doctors as by practitioners of alternative therapies, which only

A radionic practitioner using a pendulum and 'black box'
to diagnose and treat distant patients

served to convince the doctors all the more firmly that the whole business was quackery. In the United States, manufacturers of radionic equipment derived from Abrams' ideas were prosecuted and ridiculed. Ruth Drown, a chiropractor who made black boxes and a radionic 'camera' which was claimed to photograph patients' insides at a distance, allowed her equipment to be tested at Chicago University. The equipment failed to substantiate her claims for it, and Ruth Drown was later convicted and imprisoned for quackery, and all her black boxes were destroyed by Food and Drug Administration agents in 1951. She died shortly after her release from prison.

In Britain, unorthodox practitioners are not vigorously persecuted as they tend to be in the United States of America. Under common law anyone, qualified or unqualified, may practise any kind of therapy they like. There are some restrictions: you are not allowed to claim that you are medically qualified when you are not; you are not allowed to dispense drugs which are available only by doctor's prescription; you are not allowed to set yourself up as a professional surgeon; and you may not advertise treatment or cures for certain diseases, which include cancer, arthritis, glaucoma, locomotor ataxia and diabetes.

As a result of the relatively liberal laws in this country, practitioners of unusual therapies such as radionics continue to practise unmolested. Radionics tends to be a target for mocking journalists, who present the practitioner with spoof symptoms or a lock of animal fur and are provided with wildly inaccurate diagnoses of their condition. Radionics has also attracted some very dubious operators; one manufacturer of radionic instruments ran a profitable sideline selling spurious diplomas and academic qualifications. He did not, however, belong to the Radionic Association, a small organisation representing some one hundred radionic practitioners, which tries to impose ethical standards on this alternative therapy.

Radionic practitioners today have largely abandoned Dr Abrams' idea that disease emits electromagnetic radio waves, though they still use black boxes. The patient's 'witness' (for example, a lock of hair, a photograph, or a blood spot) is placed on the machine and the practitioner turns a series of dials until he or she feels a slight resistance, which indicates that the machine is tuned in to the patient. To treat the patient, the dials are placed on a setting which is calculated to correct any imbalance which may have been revealed by the radionic diagnosis. The machine is then switched to 'broadcast' healing energy to the patient.

A radionic instrument would make very little sense to a conventional electrician, who would be baffled by the fact that much of the equipment was alleged to work without being connected to any power supply. But radionic practitioners point out that the machine is just a sophisticated version of a dowser's rod, allowing them to tune in to the 'subtle energies' of the distant patient. 'Our machines do nothing that the practitioner cannot do with his own dowsing and healing faculties,' one practitioner told me. 'It is merely a tool, not the cure.'

Indeed, radionics is said to treat the patient's non-physical, spiritual energies rather than the physical body. In his book *Fringe Medicine*, Brian Inglis relates an anecdote of a patient who died while being treated radionically. His radionic practitioner had not heard about his death and pronounced him much better the next time she performed her radionic analysis. When she was told that the patient was in fact dead, she was not in the least put out: she pointed out that he was doubtless in a better place and feeling much better for it!

I have interviewed patients who claim that they had benefited from radionic therapy and could even tell when the distant radionic machine was broadcasting healing energy to them. Sadly, however, there is little in the way of documented scientific studies of the effect – or lack of effect – of radionics on large groups of patients. We have to rely on the accounts of the practitioners and their patients.

2 Placebos and self-healing

Healing, distant healing and dowsing all appear to rely on some force or energy unknown to the physicist. Traditional acupuncture and homoeopathy also appear to rely on such phenomena. But before we proceed with our tour of the outer limits of scientific speculation, let us come down to earth.

It is a fact that many people will respond well to any form of therapy they receive. When doctors arrange clinical trials to test the efficacy of a particular drug or procedure, they like to include in their study a group of patients who either receive no therapy at all or a sham therapy. If a drug is being tested, this group of patients would be given a tablet which looked like the drug in question but which really contained some medicinally inert substance like salt or sugar. This dummy therapy is called a placebo, from the Latin word meaning 'I shall please'.

Amazingly enough, a sizeable proportion of patients in any trial respond well to the placebo. From trials of pain-killing drugs, for instance, it has been found that, in general, one patient in three given the placebo will experience good pain relief and even temporary subsidence of physical symptoms such as swelling and inflammation. The placebo response tends to wear off after a few weeks, but it is real enough while it lasts. Obviously, the point of including a placebo group of patients in a clinical trial is to see whether the medicine actually works any better than the patient's faith that anything the doctor gives him must be going to do him good.

In our third programme, Dr Frank Dudley Hart spoke about one of his experiences of the placebo effect. In 1950, there had been a great deal of publicity about cortisone and its excellent effects against pain and inflammation. At about the same time, two Swedish doctors had been testing a quite different hormone preparation mixed with vitamin C, which was subsequently shown to be quite useless as a therapy for arthritis. Dr Dudley Hart let it be known that he was going to try a new drug on some of his arthritic patients, and although he in fact planned to use this Swedish preparation, the word got out among his patients that they were going to get the new wonder drug cortisone. Patients eagerly volunteered for the treatment, and some of them experienced dramatic results from it. Shortly after receiving his injection, one patient with arthritis in his hands and legs brandished his arms in the air, ran up and down the ward and jumped over his bed. 'Look, doctor,' he exclaimed, 'I haven't done this for ten years!' Dr Dudley Hart recalls the eventual outcome of this experiment:

'We later discovered that the injection we had given him had no effect on rheumatoid arthritis at all, and that this man's response was just a placebo reaction. He was so convinced that magic was on the way that it acted like magic for him. But when we repeated the experiment, the results were not half as good the next time, and soon fizzled out altogether.'

Arthritis is one of the complaints commonly taken to alternative practitioners. Dr Dudley Hart once made a confidential survey of his patients, asking them in a questionnaire to say whether they had sought alternative medical help and what results they had got from it. He found that half of the 180 patients questioned had been to an alternative practitioner or used a folklore therapy, such as wearing copper bangles. In his opinion only a few actually benefited from alternative medical ministrations, and those were mostly patients with osteoarthritis who found that osteopaths could ease the pain in their joints by gentle manipulation. Some of the folklore therapies and superstitions he has encountered in various parts of the world are scarcely believable:

'An old whale was washed up on the beach when I was in Australia, and it died and began to rot. But various members of the local population had walked inside the whale's body into its chest and some of them claimed that – unpleasant though this was in many ways – their arthritis got very much better as a result. There was also a tale told about an old tortoise, which could cure your backache if you sat on its shell.'

In Ireland there is a traditional remedy for arthritis which consists of burying the patient in manure. Dr Dudley Hart points out that this may be useful because it subjects the patient to heat, and heat can be very effective at relieving pain.

One of the aims of a clinical trial is to find out which part of a therapy achieves the desired result. For example, even if Irish manure therapy is highly effective, it is important to know whether it is the dung itself or the mere heat of the dung which is relieving the pain – otherwise patients would continue to be buried in manure when they could just as well be treated with an infra-red lamp! Alternative therapies are sometimes difficult to assess because the individual practitioner may combine, say, manipulation with diet and acupuncture treatment. If the patient improves it is hard to say which of the three treatments was responsible or, indeed, whether it was a result of combining the treatments. The doctors in Liverpool who observed the healer Bruce MacManaway at work could not determine in their short study whether the small success he did achieve was the result of his laying on of hands, his personal charm and bedside manner or the fact that he sometimes used simple manipulative techniques as well.

Dr Colin Brewer, a psychiatrist, points out that many diseases respond to suggestion and attention. One of the widely used treatments in his speciality is electro-convulsant therapy (ECT), which, despite the controversial publicity that it has attracted in recent years, is valued by many psychiatrists for its effect on depressed patients. Dr Brewer has found, however, that some depressed patients get better after being given placebo ECT. All he did was to have the patient anaesthetised as if they were going to be given ECT, but he did not actually give them the electric shock. However, he concludes 'I don't say that this proves that all the effects attributed to ECT are due to placebo, because I still believe that some patients are helped by a therapeutically induced convulsion. Nevertheless, for others it works simply because they are getting medical attention'.

A placebo effect may not just convince a patient that he is getting good therapy; it can also persuade an enthusiastic therapist that his therapy is effective, whereas the effect is really due to nature and the patient's faith. The aim of a scientifically conducted clinical trial, says Dr Brewer, should not be to prove that something works. 'You should start with the assumption that it does not work until the evidence suggests otherwise.'

Not everybody would agree with Dr Brewer's belief in the value of clinical trials. Many people, including doctors, alternative practitioners and even patients, have declared that clinical trials are unethical if they require a patient to take a placebo or do without treatment for a period of time when they could be getting an apparently effective treatment. Dr Brewer gives the counter-argument to this opinion:

'Even if you do deprive a patient of this treatment, it may transpire that you are depriving him of a treatment which in the long term proves to be harmful rather than beneficial.'

One of the other problems of clinical trials is that they are often far from conclusive. It is not uncommon for medical journals to publish one study suggesting that a therapy is effective, only for it to be followed a few weeks or months later by another study claiming the opposite. The controversy about the use of vitamin C against the common cold is a case in point. If the scientists involved are all reporting their findings accurately, where does the truth lie? Dr Brewer is not lost for an answer:

'We live in an imperfect world and the clinical trial reflects some of those imperfections. I do not think you should assume that doctors conducting clinical trials always do tell the truth. Sometimes what is known in the trade as "data massage" takes place: you succumb to the temptation to modify the data a little bit, to make an allowance here, an adjustment there, in order to produce a result which you personally would like to see. So although I say that clinical trials are important, one does not necessarily attach too much importance to a single clinical trial. The first thing scientific doctors do if somebody comes up with a report saying that a new treatment is effective is to repeat the study themselves. That is how sceptical medicine has become, and rightly so. The history of medicine is largely the history of good ideas which did not work out in practice.'

Alternative practitioners are therefore faced with a considerable task if they want to persuade a sceptical medical profession that their therapies are any good. Clinical trials are difficult enough to conduct in a large hospital or university department which is provided with staff, statisticians and computers to assess the evidence emerging from a trial involving many patients. Most alternative practitioners work in single-handed private practice and scarcely have the resources to conduct such studies. And even if they did complete clinical trials which showed that their treatment was useful, they have no guarantee of being believed or having their study published in a widely read medical journal. One of my interviewees, the naturopath and osteopath Michael van Straten, told me that he had conducted proper scientific studies of a number of herbal medicines.

One of these studies was accepted for publication by a British medical journal but rejected at the last minute by the editor, who had decided that papers about this kind of product were 'not suitable' for inclusion in the journal. He did succeed in getting other papers published, but not in journals which are widely read by the kind of doctors he would have most liked to read them.

Like many other naturopaths, Michael van Straten believes that a 'whole-food' diet which excludes meat and stimulants such as coffee can often bring great relief to people suffering from arthritis and other chronic diseases. When I asked him whether it would not be worth doing some clinical trials to substantiate this claim he replied:

'If you can find any hospital or clinical service who would be prepared to undertake clinical trials of this sort, I would be only too delighted to take part. But if you suggest such things to most consultant surgeons or physicians, they laugh at you. They are just not interested. If, on the other hand, a large pharmaceutical company were to come along with its new product and offer to spend a lot of money providing the hospital with research assistants or perhaps endow a professional chair in the university, they would fall over backwards to try the product.'

This alternative practitioner's lament is a criticism based on personal experience. But the pharmaceutical companies certainly do have very close ties with the medical profession. The food, drink and much of the organisation of the great majority of medical conferences are paid for by drug houses, and so is most of the clinical research done in hospitals. Apart from the Medical Research Council and the large charities which support research into major diseases such as cancer, there are few other sources of research funds for orthodox therapies, let alone unorthodox ones.

Fortunately, government funds have recently been made available for research into back pain, which is treated by many alternative practitioners, especially osteopaths and chiropractors. In 1979, a Department of Health working party on back pain recommended that clinical trials of manipulative therapies were urgently required, and the Department of Health has agreed to finance them.

This discussion of clinical trials has taken us away from our original topic, placebos. The point of the digression was to illustrate how doctors try to find out whether a therapy is more potent than the healing power of nature alone. The placebo is one way in which nature, aided by the human imagination, can make people feel better – or, indeed, get better physically. The disadvantage of the placebo is that its effects tend to wear off quite quickly. Admittedly, there are people who go along to their practitioner every week for harmless tonics, which do very little for their physical condition but which satisfy a need for reassurance. This kind of placebo is not so much a cure as a psychological crutch.

More serious attempts are being made to harness the self-healing power contained in a placebo, and to give it longer lasting benefits. Most of this work is being pioneered by doctors, but it fits into our definition of alternative medicine because it is intended to provide an alternative to drugs.

Dr Malcolm Carruthers, who includes among his techniques biofeedback, autogenic training and meditation, is one doctor who thought that such alternatives were necessary. 'The main difference between these techniques and drug medicine is that the patient learns how to regulate his own body rather than waiting for a pill to do it for him,' Dr Carruthers explains.

Biofeedback

Biofeedback therapy involves the use of machines which monitor the activity of physical functions such as heart rate, muscle contractions and the electrical conductivity of the skin. This information is fed back to the patient, who can then be taught how to gain control over the functions in question. In the last chapter, I described how Maxwell Cade used EEG machines to monitor brain-waves. He has found that people can quickly be taught to relax and get into meditative states with the help of an EEG. They begin by doing simple relaxation and meditation exercises, which help to slow their brain rhythms from the fast beta rhythm to the slower alpha rhythm. This change is shown on the EEG, and tells the trainee meditator that he is on the right track. The more he practises, the easier it becomes for him to induce the alpha rhythms, with the EEG acting like a mirror reflecting his progress to the relaxed state he seeks. Certainly, meditation and relaxation can be taught without the help of a machine, but biofeedback researchers claim that the machine is a useful aid for learning. As Dr Elmer Green, the American biofeedback specialist, told me: 'People who would be reluctant to believe a teacher who told them they could alter their mental state are often quite prepared to believe such things if they can be demonstrated on a machine.'

'Alpha feedback' – teaching people to induce alpha brain rhythms, has been used widely in the United States to help patients suffering from migraine and tension headaches. There has been

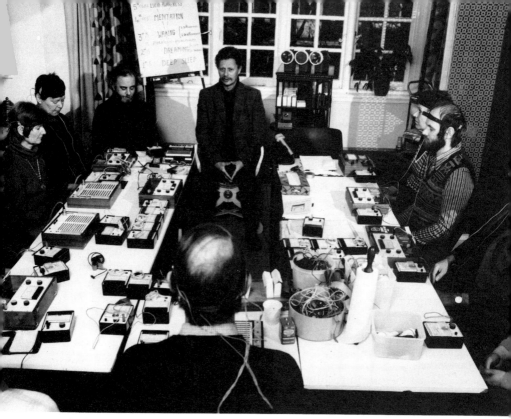

*A biofeedback class learning to regulate their brain
activity through relaxation and meditation*

some controversy about the need for the biofeedback machines, with some therapists claiming that biofeedback is really no more effective in the long term than simple relaxation exercises. But the biofeedback buffs maintain that results can be obtained more rapidly when the patient has a machine to reflect how he is doing.

A simpler form of biofeedback used to help sufferers from migraine consists of hand-warming exercises. The patient is provided with a little thermometer, costing just a few pence, which is taped to his hand. He is then shown how he can raise the temperature of his hand just by relaxing and imagining that the hand is getting warmer. To someone who has not tried it, this may sound too incredibly simple to be true. In fact, most people can manage it at their first lesson. The trick is not aggressively to will your hand to get warmer (this often achieves the reverse effect) but calmly say to yourself, 'My hand is getting warmer.' Children can usually learn this technique very quickly, according to Dr Elmer Green. Youngsters he has taught have been able to raise the temperature of one hand several degrees higher than that of the other at the first or second attempt.

The apparent reason why hand warming helps migraine sufferers is that it gives them some control over their sympathetic nervous system. This is the system which stimulates the flow of blood in major arteries during moments of stress. As some migraine headaches are caused by an excessive flow of blood to the head, a technique which helps to check this surge should also succeed in reducing headaches.

Another biofeedback technique can help people with high blood pressure. Small electrodes are taped to the fingers, and attached to a device which monitors the electrical conductivity of the skin. The conductivity of the skin reflects arousal, stress or nervousness. Very briefly, when you are relaxed, your hands tend to be dry and their electrical conductivity is low. When you are aroused or nervous, your hands tend to become damper and their electrical conductivity increases. Another effect of arousal or stress is increased blood pressure. Therefore, a London doctor, Chandra Patel, reasoned that if patients could be taught how to reduce the electrical conductivity of their skin they might also be able to reduce their high blood pressure.

The machine used by Dr Patel has a dial which gives a reading on the skin conductivity, and it is also provided with a little loudspeaker, which emits a variable tone. As you become nervous and aroused, the tone rises higher; as you relax, the tone falls; and when you become very relaxed and the conductivity of the skin on your hands is reduced, the tone disappears altogether. Dr Patel would explain the machine to her patients and teach them to relax physically by listening to taped relaxation exercises or by simple yoga. She has now published several papers in The Lancet and other medical journals reporting how biofeedback and relaxation helped the great majority of her patients to reduce their high blood pressure to such an extent that most of them were able to give up or significantly reduce the amount of drugs they had previously had to take to keep their blood pressure under control. In one study she conducted with Dr Malcolm Carruthers, they found that the therapy could also help cigarette smokers to reduce their smoking and even bring down the level of cholesterol in the blood. Cholesterol is a kind of fat, and high levels of cholesterol in the blood are often found in people with heart disease. Heart specialists have recommended that people who want to avoid heart disease should not let their cholesterol level get too high, and they have generally suggested that the best way to ensure this is to avoid eating eggs and foods rich in animal fats. But Patel and Carruthers' studies suggest that relaxation and stress control may be just as effective.

Autogenic training

Autogenic training could be described as biofeedback without the instruments. 'One of the drawbacks of biofeedback,' Dr Carruthers says, 'is that part of your attention is always directed away from yourself to the machine, wondering what the box of tricks is up to. With autogenic training all your attention is directed inside yourself. You could regard it as a Western form of meditation.'

In practice and principle, autogenic training looks even more simple than biofeedback. The basis of the training is to get the patient to repeat phrases suggesting that particular parts of the body are becoming heavy and warm. This can induce deep relaxation and the resolution of many complaints which are brought on or aggravated by stress and psychosomatic disturbances.

A typical session might begin with the trainees lying out flat on mattresses or easy chairs. The therapist begins by telling them to relax, close their eyes and breathe slowly and deeply. They are then told to repeat, slowly, gently and in their own time, suggestive phrases such as 'My arms feel heavy and warm,' 'My legs feel heavy and warm,' 'My forehead is cool,' 'My heartbeat is calm and regular,' 'My mind is quiet and happy,' or 'I am still and at peace.' Each phrase might be repeated several times, and the therapist may take the trainees on a tour of their body, getting them to imagine each limb feeling heavy and warm and each organ functioning smoothly and quietly.

Autogenic training is a relatively new therapy to Britain, but it has a long history. In 1910, a French pharmacist, Emil Coué, invented a simple technique for people whom he thought would benefit more from a medicine for their minds than a conventional prescription. He suggested that they should say to themselves, 'Every day and in every way I am feeling better and better.' The term 'autogenics' was coined by a German doctor, Johannes Schultz, in the 1920s. He, too, believed that relaxation was often the best therapy, and he used hypnosis to make his patients relax. But he had two objections to hypnosis. Although it worked very well on some people, there were others who could not be hypnotised. They resisted the hypnotist's attempts to lull them into trance. His second objection to hypnosis was that the hypnotist was essentially manipulating a passive patient. Schultz thought that for relaxation therapy to work best, the patient should be relaxing himself rather than relying on a hypnotist to do it for him.

Since the 1920s, autogenic training has been quite widely applied in Europe and the United States, and there are hundreds of reports in the medical literature attesting to its value in the treatment of diseases which are due, partly or wholly, to the effects of stress. Asthma, high blood pressure, migraine, anxiety and, sometimes, skin diseases like eczema and psoriasis have often responded well to autogenic training. John Gold, one of the patients interviewed for our programmes, had had a long history of nervous depression and insomnia, for which he had taken a variety of tranquillisers and sleeping pills. After a course of eight week-end sessions of autogenic training, he claimed that he 'could now sleep like the proverbial log' and had given up all his drugs.

Unlike a surgical operation or a course of antibiotics, autogenic training does not claim to provide a once-and-for-all solution to a problem. Having learnt it, the trainee may need to practise it regularly, or at least at moments when the stresses and strains which lay at the root of his problem threaten to engulf him again.

'Whenever I start to feel nervous or under pressure or can't sleep,' John Gold says, 'I go through the autogenic routine, imagining my arms feeling heavy and warm and so on, and a wonderful warm feeling comes over me and I feel content and relaxed.'

Despite its apparent simplicity and safety, autogenic training can present problems requiring the help of an experienced therapist. Dr Carruthers has found, for instance, that trainees in a state of deep relaxation sometimes recall distressing events from their earlier life or even feel pain from old and apparently healed injuries. Re-experiencing these old traumas, he says, is an important part of the training, allowing the trainee to release pent-up feelings which may be contributing to his stress.

Carruthers believes that the great value of therapies like biofeedback and autogenic training is that they harness the mind and body's self-healing resources:

'The body does have enormous recuperative and restorative powers. After researching for some ten years into the many and varied effects of stress, I

feel that a lot of conventional medicines, while they help in some respects, can impair these self-healing and self-balancing systems. I think it is virtually impossible to use a drug regime to get all the body's complex and various systems back into adjustment in the long term.'

Other mental therapies

Carruthers therefore sees non-drug therapies such as autogenic training as a genuine alternative in the treatment of 'mind-made' diseases. But can we draw a line between diseases which are aggravated by psychological stress and those in which the mind plays no part at all? Another of our interviewees, Dr Ian Pearce, believes not:

'Most disease is what we have created within us, either through our mental or emotional processes or through misbehaviour in terms of looking after our bodies properly, by eating poor diets, working in bad environments, following wrong life styles. It is only when you get these things right that you can begin to encourage the body's powers of self-healing.'

Dr Pearce, a Norfolk GP, is primarily interested in using self-healing techniques in the treatment of cancer. He believes that in many cases cancer is a psychosomatic disease, in which the physical functioning of the body has been upset by disturbed mental and emotional processes. This is still a highly controversial approach, but one which is beginning to attract serious attention from doctors. Several experienced cancer specialists have suggested that people who are prone to depression or, more especially, tend to suppress their emotions are at greater risk of dying from cancer. They have found that people who respond with a 'fighting spirit' when they are told they have cancer are more likely to overcome the illness or survive a longer time than people who quickly give up hope.

In 1967, the American cancer specialist Dr D. Kissen made a psychological comparison of a group of smokers who had lung cancer with smokers of similar age and status who did not have the disease. He found that the smokers with lung cancer were more liable to deny or repress their emotions. Another study by Dr D. W. Abse and his colleagues in 1974 revealed that lung cancer patients who smoke tend to be less-assertive than smokers in general. More recently, Dr Steven Greer and his colleagues at King's College Hospital Medical School in London have studied women with breast cancer. They discovered through questioning the women and their families that breast cancer was often associated with a life-long tendency to suppress emotions, particularly anger. They also found that this psychological characteristic was associated with changes in the immune system, the body's defence mechanism against disease. They noticed that the women who suppressed their anger tended to have in their blood higher levels of a substance called serum IgA, and that there was good evidence that this could contribute to the growth of tumours.

An editorial in *The Lancet* (31 March 1979), entitled 'Mind and Cancer', summarised this research and several other studies which had suggested that cancer patients who had a strong will to live did indeed live longer than those who felt helpless in the face of the disease. One of the doctors whose work was quoted, Dr Ainsley Meares of Australia, has found that his patients could be helped by learning to meditate, and has documented several striking case histories in which large tumours have regressed after the patient began meditating. The American radiotherapist, Dr Carl Simonton of Fort Worth, Texas, has had similar success with another mental therapy. He encourages his patients to imagine that their tumours are being overcome by the body's immune forces. One way in which he might do this is to suggest that the patient pictures the cancer cells as Western outlaws dressed in black and the healthy cells of the immune system as good cowboys dressed in white, surrounding and shooting down the black outlaws. *The Lancet* cautiously pointed out that it was still uncertain whether these therapies which encouraged patients to 'fight back' worked by a placebo effect or by activating more profound self-healing mechanisms. But 'whether or not dynamic hope or "fighting back" will prolong life in the cancer patient beyond its expected duration, it is almost certain that absence of hope can shorten life, apart from vitiating its quality,' the editorial commented.

The doctors who use these mental therapies regard them as supplementary rather than alternative to orthodox cancer therapy. Dr Simonton, for instance, still gives his patients radiotherapy for their tumours as well as teaching them his 'creative visualisation' technique. Dr Ian Pearce takes a similar line. He teaches his patients creative visualisation and biofeedback, which he combines with laying on of hands by a healer and dietary advice. 'But I must make it plain,' he says, 'that I do not advocate this as an alternative to ordinary methods of therapy. It is complementary rather than alternative, indeed I deprecate the use of the word "alternative".'

Dr Pearce was motivated to seek complementary methods of treating cancer after his only daughter had died from leukaemia in 1966.

Although modern drugs, surgery and radiotherapy really have improved the prospects of people suffering from certain types of cancer, he realised that many forms of the disease were still quite incurable, and that the conventional treatments often exacted an unpleasant toll in side effects without improving the length of the patient's life, let alone its quality. One of his aims is to help his patients improve what might be called the 'inner quality' of their daily lives:

'The therapy involves teaching the patient a discipline of deep relaxation of mind and body, calming the emotions, centring of the mind and then retiring into a sort of inner sanctum of peace and tranquillity, so that their level of stress and arousal is minimal. They are then asked to, as it were, turn their eyes within them and try to make a journey through their body, visualising the disease process and trying to see what it is doing to them in terms of causing pain, loss of appetite or whatever their predominant symptoms are. Then they are asked to look a little further and see that the body has its own defensive cells in the immune system whose function it is to destroy and discharge unhealthy tissue and unhealthy cells. They are asked to visualise that they are in control of this process and to see the immune system's cells swarming around and attacking the tumour. They are encouraged to see the tumour not as something very large and firm and rigid, but as something rather shapeless, composed of cells which have, as it were, lost their way. We ask them to do this about three times a day for a period of about fifteen minutes, and we supplement that with fortnightly group sessions which are conducted as a kind of miniature healing service, involving prayer, music, meditation and, once they are in a state of deep relaxation, laying on of hands.'

Dr Pearce makes no claims that his complementary therapy has cured any of his patients. Firstly, he has only been doing this work with a small number of patients for a few years. Secondly, almost all his patients have already received or are still receiving conventional treatment. However, he does claim that his patients tend to respond better to the conventional treatment they get than might otherwise be expected. Unpleasant symptoms such as pain, lethargy, loss of appetite, depression and sleeplessness tend to ease. And he believes that many of the patients who come to him when they are already at death's door overcome their feelings of distress and helplessness in the face of death.

Even though Meares, Simonton and Pearce all have reports of individual patients who responded well to mental self-healing, it would be difficult to perform clinical trials to prove whether such complementary therapy worked consistently or to demonstrate whether particular types of people were better at self-healing than others. As *The Lancet*'s editorial pointed out: 'Patients would need to be stratified according to their beliefs, intelligence and temperament, apart from type and stage of cancer, and such a trial seems hardly feasible in our present state of knowledge.' This type of therapy is time-consuming, and calls for a devoted practitioner who can work with only a small number of patients at any one time. Much more than with drugs, surgery and radiotherapy, its success must depend on the skill of the practitioner in persuading the patient that he wants to get better and in the patient's belief that this can be done.

3 Acupuncture

The first chapter of this book spoke of extraordinary, inexplicable skills and energies. In the second chapter I tried to show that feats of self-healing were, if not ordinary, at least well within the normal capabilities of the human being. Acupuncture combines the extraordinary with the normal. On the one hand, it is alleged to stimulate a 'vital energy' which is said to run along invisible channels. On the other hand, it can to a certain extent be explained in terms of conventional anatomy, and it can be practised by people without extraordinary psychic talents or healing gifts.

Acupuncture in China

I had better start with a very brief explanation of the traditional Chinese theory behind acupuncture. This theory may not make sense to anyone acquainted with Western ideas of anatomy and physiology, but it is the rationale of traditional acupuncture. Even though some Western practitioners of acupuncture do not believe in the ancient theory, and even though doctors in the People's Republic of China largely reject it too, nearly all of them have learnt it and still find that its doctrines can be useful in practice.

Traditional Chinese medicine sees man very much as part of his environment, and describes health as being in harmony with the elements and energies of that environment. The essence of harmony is the balance of Yin and Yang. Yin and Yang cannot really be described as elements or energies. They are more like our ideas of negative and positive, female and male. 'Dynamic states' might be one way to describe them. The earth, moon, winter, water, the valley and the female are said to be Yin, while the male Yang is said to be present in the sun, summer, heaven, fire and the mountain top.

There are five elements: water, wood, fire, earth and metal, said to be the basis of all matter. And there is the vital energy, *Chi* (pronounced 'key'), which quickens all living matter and whose vigour, flow and distribution depends on a proper balance of the elements and Yin and Yang.

Chi is said to circulate around the body along channels or meridians. Whether or not these channels exist in any physical way is the subject of debate between traditional and modern theorists, but it is along these meridians that the many points used for needling are situated. There are twelve principal meridians, ten of which are associated with particular organs of the body and two of which correspond to 'functions'. The Yin organs tend to be the solid ones: liver, heart, spleen, kidney and lungs; whereas the Yang organs are hollow: stomach, bladder, gall bladder, large intestine, small intestine. The function associated with circulation and sexuality, is Yin; while the other, called *sanjiao* or 'the triple warmer', is Yang. There are another two important meridians: the 'conception vessel', which runs from the perineum to the chin along the front of the body, and the 'governing vessel', which runs down the spine.

The job of the acupuncturist is to ensure that *Chi* flows along these channels at the proper rate. He diagnoses the condition of each organ, either by looking at the tongue and examining its colour and coating or by taking the pulse. The way in which the Chinese take the pulse is considerably more complex than the Western method of just feeling the strength and speed of the blood flowing through the radial artery at the wrist. Each of the invisible meridians passes through the wrist, six on the right hand and six on the left. The pulse of each meridian is felt by pressing either lightly or deeply at various points on the radial artery, and the experienced acupuncturist is supposed to be able to detect up to twenty-eight different qualities in each pulse, which indicate to him how well the vital energy is flowing.

Having discovered from this pulse diagnosis which organ or organs are working too hard or too feebly, the acupuncturist will insert his needles at given points along the corresponding meridian. The point where the needle is inserted may have no obvious connection in conventional Western anatomical terms with the part of the body which is causing the patient trouble. For instance, the acupuncturist may see migraine as a disturbance of liver function, and insert his needle in the point known as Liver 3, which lies between the big and second toes! Acupuncture points can also be

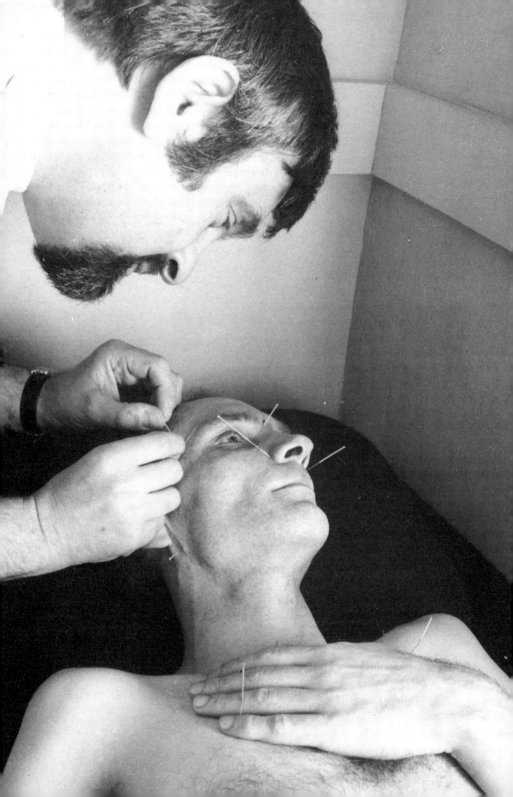

stimulated by pressing on them with a thumb (this is known as acupressure or Shiatsu), or by heating them with smouldering cones of the herb mugwort, *Artemesia moxa*. Moxibustion, as this technique is called, does not actually burn the skin because the herb is removed before it burns too far down. Sometimes the moxa is burned in a little cradle on top of a needle so that its heat passes through the needle into the skin.

One might well ask how the Chinese came to devise such a theory and practice. The history of acupuncture goes back some 2,500 years, and one can only assume that it derived from centuries of observation and speculation. It is known that doctors in Africa and Arabia as well as China used stone, wooden or metal needles or thorns many centuries ago to relieve pain or to drain the pus from wounds.

Acupuncture in the West

Acupuncture was brought to Europe in the last century by Jesuit missionaries who had travelled in China and the East. Although most people believe that acupuncture is a new therapy in the West, doctors have in fact used needles to relieve pain for many years. In 1912, for instance, the famous physician Sir William Osler in his textbook *Principles and Practice of Medicine* recommended 'ordinary bonnet needles, sterilised . . . and thrust into the lumbar muscles' as the most efficient treatment for lumbago.

Pain is the commonest reason for the use of acupuncture in the West, though it is employed for treating almost every complaint in China, Korea and Taiwan. Acupuncturists here have recently claimed that their therapy can successfully treat addictions, asthma, infertility and even baldness. A recent paper in the *Chinese Medical Journal* reported how doctors there had found it useful for relieving the symptoms of malaria. In the East, however, acupuncture is seldom used alone. Chinese medicine covers many therapies: herbs, diet, massage and meditation, and no doctor or even 'barefoot doctor' would be allowed to practise if he only knew the technique of sticking in needles.

When we talk about pain, we should distinguish between *preventing* pain and *relieving* pain. It is necessary to prevent pain during a surgical operation; ability to tolerate pain has to be increased before the painful procedures actually begin. Analgesic acupuncture can be effective, though it seems that some people respond much better to it than others. Ten years ago, the majority of surgical patients in

47

Chinese hospitals used to be given acupuncture analgesia (often in addition to doses of normal anaesthetic drugs). Today, only a small minority have acupuncture as their only analgesic, and these tend to be those who are known to respond well.

Acupuncture analgesia is used in this country by doctors to help patients through dental surgery or childbirth. Its main disadvantage is that it can take up to twenty minutes of twiddling the needles to raise the patient's pain tolerance, and it needs to be continued throughout the operation. It may be a useful addition to conventional anaesthetics – indeed, it has been used in more than 1,200 operations at the German Heart Centre in Munich to reduce the amount of drugs given to anaesthetised patients – but the operating theatre is not likely to be the main place where we shall see acupuncture practised.

Acupuncture will probably prove to be most useful in relieving pain. Specialists in many National Health Service hospital pain clinics now include acupuncture in the battery of treatments they try on patients with back-aches, migraines, rheumatic pains and neuralgias which fail to respond to drugs or surgery. In his book *The Control of Chronic Pain*, one of Britain's most experienced pain specialists, Dr Sampson Lipton, writes about acupuncture:

'It can be used as a non-invasive simple method of relieving pain. In the author's experience it is particularly useful in chronic migraine patients who do not respond to the normal treatments available; after they have been fully investigated to exclude neurological disease, acupuncture will produce relief in about two-thirds of them to the extent of a reduction of two thirds in both the pain and the frequency of attacks. There will, of course, be some patients whose migraine is completely relieved and a few patients whose migraine appears to be made worse.'

How does it work?

However, what we still want to know is how a needle inserted into your foot can relieve a headache. Those who follow the traditional theory are not at a loss for an explanation: it is due to stimulation of *Chi* along the liver meridian. Western anatomists who have seen migraine treated this way refuse to accept the existence of meridians and *Chi*, but are still unable to explain the phenomenon on their own scientific terms.

There are some ways in which the effects of acupuncture can be explained by Western scientific knowledge and theory. Firstly, many traditional acupuncture points are situated at places where small bundles of nerves emerge from the deeper tissue towards the surface of the body. If these nerves are stimulated – and they can be stimulated by massage, heat, ice or gentle electric currents as well as by a needle – the signals they transmit to the brain have the effect of blotting out the weaker signals from other nerves which are telling the brain that it should be feeling pain.

'We also know,' says Dr David Bowsher, the Liverpool University anatomist, 'that if you "block" the nerves with a local anaesthetic, acupuncture does not work. This suggests that the mechanism with which we are dealing is in the nerves and not due to some mysterious energy.'

Recent research also suggests that acupuncture analgesia may be due in part to substances called endorphins. Endorphins were first discovered in 1975. They are chemicals (long chains of peptides, to be more exact) which are produced by the pituitary gland and have a similar effect to morphine, in so far as they appear to relieve pain and change mood. Though the endorphins are not similar in their chemical structure to morphine, they attach themselves to the same receptors in the brain and gut to which morphine has to attach itself to exert its effect. Endorphins are released, together with other pituitary hormones, during moments of stress, and it now seems that the reason soldiers or sportsmen can sometimes put up with severe injuries during conflict without feeling pain at the time is that their pituitary gland is pumping out pain-killing endorphins. The Swedish pharmacologist Professor Lars Terenius of Uppsala University has found that endorphins are released into the spinal fluid when the body is given acupuncture-like stimulation. Several researchers, including Professor Terenius and Dr Bowsher, have noticed that the pain-killing effects of acupuncture can be nullified if the patient is given a drug called naloxone. This drug is an opiate antagonist, which means that it counteracts the effects of opiate drugs like morphine and the natural opiates like endorphins by dislodging them from their receptors in the brain. So, if acupuncture analgesia can be abolished by naloxone, it is reasonable to conclude that the analgesia was originally caused by endorphins.

It is worth noting at this point that hypnotic analgesia is not affected by naloxone. Hypnosis can be very effective at preventing pain and has been used, like acupuncture, to get people through operations, dental surgery and childbirth without painkilling drugs. Sceptics have often claimed that acupuncture is no more than a form of hypnosis or suggestion, and with such a dramatic therapy as acupuncture the placebo element may indeed be substantial. Nevertheless, there are obvious physiological differences between acupuncture analgesia and hypnotic analgesia. For one thing, hypnotic analgesia does not involve the endorphins.

Endorphins can provide only a partial explanation, however. Acupuncture pain relief is sometimes very fast, certainly a lot quicker than anything that could be achieved by the release of endorphins, which may take twenty minutes or more to reach significant levels in the central nervous system.

Western medicine and traditional acupuncture bear each other out in another phenomenon – trigger points. Trigger points are mysterious: nobody knows exactly how they are caused. Nevertheless, they are very commonly found in people suffering from pain. A trigger point is a tender spot which usually occurs quite near the painful area, though it can occur some distance away. A well-known trigger point is 'McBurney's point', a tender spot on the abdomen which occurs in appendicitis. People with heart conditions often have trigger points in their shoulder, chest or arm. If a trigger point is poked, it will be sore or send a stab of pain to the damaged organ. Strangely, though, if it is more vigorously stimulated with a needle, heat or electric current or injected with a local anaesthetic, the pain in the affected organ will diminish or disappear. The pain researcher Professor Ronald Melzack of McGill University has compared trigger points with the traditional acupuncture points used for relieving pain, and has found that they coincide to a very high degree. He has therefore come to the conclusion that, although trigger points and acupuncture pain points were discovered independently on different sides of the world and have different names, they are really the same phenomenon.

Acupuncture points

Students of acupuncture begin learning the location of the many acupuncture points by consulting charts. In the old Chinese schools they had to know these points by heart. To test their knowledge the teacher would take a small metal statue of the human body which was hollow and provided with holes where the acupuncture points were supposed to be. The statue would be covered in wax and filled with water. The student would then have to insert his needles where he thought the points were. He would know each time he was right because a little spurt of water would gush through the wax. In practice, though, acupuncture points do not occur on exactly the same spot on every body. The acupuncturist will know the approximate area of its location, but he will usually find the point itself by feeling the skin; a point needing treatment may feel slightly tough, knotty or tender. He may use an electrode needle attached to a device which measures the electrical resistance of the skin. The acupuncture point will be shown as a small area of very low resistance. The toughness or low resistance will generally disappear after the point has been needled for a few minutes.

Meridians

Although there is general agreement between East and West that acupuncture points are a genuine physical phenomenon (even though no one knows how they get there), what are we to make of the meridians? Orthodox medical opinion holds that they just do not exist. The traditional acupuncturists aver that they most certainly do, and cite studies which claim that the meridians can be traced as lines of low electrical resistance in the skin. In 1965, a North Korean medical researcher, Kim Bong Han, claimed that he had found anatomical evidence of the meridians, and amazed his Chinese colleagues with cadavers on which he had been able to trace the paths of the meridians in coloured dyes. He claimed that he could dissect the meridians and had found distinct kinds of tissue in them. The 'corpuscles of Kim Bong Han' were the talk of acupuncturists for some time. However, despite repeated attempts by Chinese scientists to duplicate Kim's work, none of them was able to find his corpuscles. His work is now widely believed to be an elaborate fraud which was deliberately encouraged by the North Korean government to steal a march on the Chinese, who were also keen to re-establish their ancient therapy in scientific terms.

Dr Richard Clark, one of the few British doctors to practise acupuncture full time, is not very worried whether meridians exist physically or not:

'For me a meridian is an idea which connects various useful points on the body. It is not an organic entity like a blood vessel or nerve. People have tried to show that meridians follow nerve pathways, but although this is sometimes true, it is not consistently true of all the main meridians.'

One reason the Chinese may have developed the idea of meridians is that people undergoing acupuncture experience sensations rather like water flowing or ants crawling. This sensation, which the Chin-

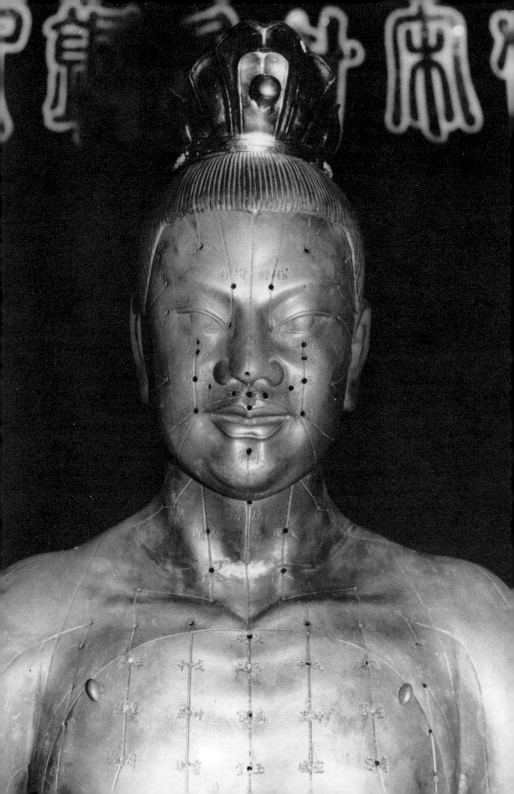

ese call *Techi*, runs in a line away from the acupuncture point which is being needled. Richard Clark's first patient gave a graphic description of this when a needle was put into his hand near his little finger:

'He said it was as though his arm was a trough of water, and that a wave was passing along one side of it into his shoulder blade. He described the same sensation in his legs when I treated a point in his foot. On both occasions this wave appeared to be running along the line of the meridian in question.'

Techi is a common sensation, and is taken by acupuncturists as a sign that they are stimulating the right spot and that the patient is likely to respond well.

Is *Techi* a manifestation of vital energy or is it some kind of reflex action of the autonomic nervous system? So far no Western scientist has come up with a complete explanation to replace the ancient Chinese one. But if you prefer to stick with the Chinese idea of *Chi*, you might well still wonder how a metal needle could have any effect on the flow of a non-physical energy.

In some respects, acupuncture has a similar effect to that of a gentle electric current. Pain specialists have found that electrical stimulation of the skin at a frequency of 1–2Hz relieves pain in the same way as acupuncture. Acupuncturists often feed a small electric current through their needles; this can be as effective as twirling the needles by hand and therefore allows the acupuncturist to treat more than one patient at a time.

When to try acupuncture

In 1979, the World Health Organisation held a symposium in Peking for medical acupuncturists from all over the world, and got them to draw up a list of diseases which lent themselves to acupuncture treatment. The list named more than forty major diseases, including sinusitis, the common cold, tonsillitis, bronchitis, asthma, eye disorders, toothache, gastritis, colitis, duodenal ulcer, constipation, diarrhoea, migraine, facial pains, nervous disorders, musculo-skeletal pains, Menière's disease and osteoarthritis. It was not claimed that acupuncture could completely cure all these complaints but that it could provide symptomatic relief.

A hollow model of the human body used by the Chinese to teach the location of acupuncture points

Acupuncture has been known to relieve individual cases of many other complaints, though responsible acupuncturists would not claim that acupuncture worked in all cases. For instance, Dr Richard Clark tells of two of his female patients who had been infertile for several years before receiving acupuncture. One of them had had one of her Fallopian tubes removed and was suffering from an ovarian cyst. She had previously had an inflammatory disease of the pelvis after a Dalkon Shield intra-uterine contraceptive device had caused an infection in her womb.

'She had been trying to conceive for a long time but had given up hope that she would ever get pregnant. She originally came for acupuncture because of the pain from her ovarian cyst and because she was fed up with orthodox treatment – which is, unfortunately, a common reason why people seek an alternative. Nine months after receiving intermittent acupuncture she became pregnant.'

Though both doctor and patient were delighted with the result, especially when she went on to have acupuncture to relieve pain during her delivery, Dr Clark admits that he cannot explain just how acupuncture helped in this case.

'The Chinese would explain it as a correction of energy balance, but it is hard to see how that could overcome such a gross mechanical problem as apparently existed in her reproductive system. But again subtle changes caused by the treatment could have tipped the balance. Possibly some sort of autonomic reflex improved the circulation of blood in her reproductive system and therefore maximised its potential. Perhaps the acupuncture set off reflexes which caused a musculo-skeletal readjustment resulting in a straightening out of her kinked Fallopian tube. But really, I just do not know.'

The risks

Sticking needles into people is obviously a procedure which is not without risk. There have been a few cases of acupuncturists giving their patients hepatitis by using unsterilized needles. Some patients have been made very ill by having long needles inserted by unskilled practitioners into their heart or lungs. A more common criticism made by doctors of non-medically qualified acupuncturists is that they can mask the symptoms of serious disease by getting rid of the patient's pain. With the pain gone, the patient happily assumes that all is well – which may be far from true.

I put this criticism to Professor Jack Worsley, who is head of the College of Traditional Chinese Acupuncture in Leamington Spa, and who is not medically qualified. (His professorship is an honorary title awarded by a university in South Korea.) He replied that he thought it was 'criminal and exceedingly dangerous' to use acupuncture simply as a means of removing painful symptoms, and ran against the traditional Chinese methods, which were aimed at treating disease at its source. But he suggested that doctors who had learnt only the rudiments of acupuncture were more guilty of this charge than those acupuncturists, not medically qualified, who had been more thoroughly trained in traditional practice. Dr Richard Clark agreed with him, commenting as a doctor that he would prefer to see patients treated by a trained acupuncturist who was not a medical doctor than by a well-qualified doctor who had learnt all his acupuncture from one week's course of instruction. And Dr Julian Kenyon, a Liverpool doctor who himself runs short courses for doctors, said that he thought that many acupuncturists who were not medically qualified were much better versed in the subject than doctors:

'I am afraid that many doctors are guilty of practising acupuncture from a book. A patient comes with, say, migraine, so he looks up which points can be used for relieving migraine and puts in his needles. This will produce results in some patients, but it will make others worse. As a doctor and acupuncturist I use both the diagnostic methods I was taught at medical school and the traditional Chinese methods. You must be able to make a correct Chinese diagnosis because that will tell you where to put your pins. If you put your pin into a point on the liver meridian when it should be on the stomach meridian, the patient will probably get worse.'

Western sceptics dismiss traditional Chinese theories as so much unintelligible hocus-pocus. Traditional practitioners such as Jack Worsley declare that acupuncture is based soundly on centuries of observation of the laws of nature, and that it will be the sceptics who will eventually have to admit that the old ideas, despite their alien-sounding concepts, were right. But as Professor Melzack found when he compared acupuncture points and trigger points, it may turn out that the controversy is due more to differences in language and philosophy than to matters of fact.

4 Homoeopathy

Homoeopathy is another therapy which seems to involve the harnessing of an energy beyond the ken of orthodox science. Though it is practised largely by doctors, it stands the basic ideas of conventional medicine on their head. The first principle of homoeopathy is that 'like cures like' – in other words, that the medicine which cures a patient contains ingredients which would actually give them the very symptoms they are complaining of. Another of its principles is that tiny doses work better than large ones. Indeed, many homoeopathic remedies have been diluted so many times that they can hardly still contain one molecule of the original ingredient.

How could anyone believe that people can be cured by giving them sub-molecular quantities of manifest poisons? Let us first take a brief look at the history of homoeopathy.

History

The originator of homoeopathy was the physician Samuel Hahnemann, who was born in Meissen, Saxony, in 1755. Dr Hahnemann was a scrupulous practitioner who regarded many of the practices of his contemporary medical colleagues as little better than licensed poisoning and butchery. Like some doctors today, he believed that many of the medicines and therapies in use at the time did more harm than good, and he set out to improve medical practice by close study of the action of drugs, which were then almost all herbal products.

In 1790, Hahnemann was experimenting with cinchona, the source of the modern medicine quinine, which was then one of the few substances which could help to control the symptoms of malaria, a disease which was quite common in Europe in those days. He was not suffering from malaria himself, but he found that when he took a hefty dose of cinchona he experienced similar symptoms to those of that disease: fever, shiveriness and rigours. (Quinine has fallen out of favour in recent years because large doses were found to cause side effects similar to those from which Hahnemann suffered.)

Firstly, he wondered whether he was abnormally sensitive to cinchona, but after trying the medicine on some of his patients he found that they reacted in the same way. He was intrigued by the fact that a drug which could relieve a disease could also, if given in large enough doses, give you the symptoms of that disease. He conceived the idea that symptoms might be a manifestation of the body's fight against disease, and that an effective medicine worked because it was helping the body in that fight.

Hahnemann had had plenty of opportunity to study at first hand the effects of overdosage from many kinds of medicine. Belladonna, for example, was a popular medicine for colic, but in overdosage it produced effects which were like the symptoms of scarlet fever. He tried treating scarlet-fever patients with safer doses of belladonna, and they responded well. Since he was now giving his patients medicines which could aggravate their symptoms, he experimented with ever smaller doses, and came to the conclusion that they were often more beneficial.

Because he wanted to have close control over the quality and quantity of medicines his patients received, Hahnemann prepared his remedies personally. In 1810, he published his book, *The Organon of Rational Healing*, describing methods of diluting and 'succussing' medicines (shaking them vigorously by hand). Prepared in this way, he claimed, remedies became 'potentised' so that tiny doses could be used safely and to good effect.

Hahnemann was popular with his patients, many of whom must have found that his medicines were less likely to do them harm than those prescribed by more heavy-handed medical men. But most doctors thought that his ideas about 'potentising' by dilution and succussion were nonsensical, and apothecaries were alarmed lest their business be adversely affected by this fashion for tiny doses. Nevertheless, his book did attract admirers who shared his concern about the side effects of contemporary medicine.

One of those admirers was the London physician Frederick Foster Quin, who went to learn from Hahnemann, and in 1850 established a hospital in London to put Hahnemann's ideas into practice. Those ideas were now known as 'homoeopathy' (from the Greek words meaning 'similar to the disease'); the homoeopaths described conventional medicine, which sought to fight against symptoms rather than work with them, as 'allopathy', which is derived from the Greek words meaning 'different from the disease'.

Quin enjoyed considerable success with the new homoeopathy, largely because he had friends in the aristocracy who spread the word in fashionable society. This aroused the jealousy of orthodox physicians, who tried unsuccessfully to have him denounced as a charlatan and barred from professional practice.

In 1854, London was ravaged by an epidemic of cholera, and this plague turned out to be a blessing in disguise for the homoeopaths. In those days most people who caught cholera died, and the mortality rate of cholera patients in the London hospitals was over fifty per cent – except at Quin's homoeopathic hospital, where the death toll was only one patient in six.

It was this early success, together with the patronage Quin enjoyed from the aristocracy, that ensured that homoeopathy became recognised as a medical speciality. Although the majority of doctors are still either ignorant of the subject (it is not taught in medical schools) or are scornful of its claims and philosophy, homoeopathy is practised in National Health Service hospitals in London, Bristol, Glasgow and Liverpool. Unlike practitioners of other alternative therapies most homoeopaths are qualified doctors. And the noble patronage continues: one of the Queen's physicians is a homoeopathic doctor.

Principles of homoeopathy

The idea of 'like curing like' is a puzzling one, but as Dr Robin Gibson, a consultant homoeopathic physician in Glasgow, points out, it is not a particularly unusual phenomenon:

'We use many substances in this manner. A hot cup of tea, for instance, will cool you more quickly on a hot day than a glass of cold water. X-rays which can produce cancer are also used curatively in the treatment of cancer. And aspirin, which in overdosage can give you a very high temperature, is used in proper therapeutic doses to reduce temperature. There is a double-sided action to all drugs, and this is something conventional medicine tends to forget.'

In conventional allopathic medicine the chosen drug is aimed at the disease process: a bacterial infection is treated with an antibiotic, inflammation with an anti-inflammatory drug. In homoeopathy, the remedy is aimed at the patient as a whole: it takes into account not just the symptoms of his or her physical illness but also character, moods, likes and dislikes and family history. The homoeopath may spend as long as an hour at the first consultation taking note of all kinds of details which may seem quite irrelevant. Does the patient dislike milk or fatty foods? Does he sweat a lot? Does she hate the damp? Is he tidy? Is she excitable or prone to burst into tears? All this information is then set against what the homoeopath knows about the effects of his medicines. From Hahnemann onwards homoeopaths have studied the effects of their medicines on volunteers, and tried to note every effect on the body, mood, diet and psyche which these medicines appeared to have had. All this material is collected in a reference book, the *Materia Medica*, and the homoeopath's skill consists in matching the individual patient with a medicine which is known to make people feel as that patient is now feeling.

Let us take influenza as an example. The allopathic doctor sees it as a single disease. The homoeopath is less interested in the diagnosis of 'flu than in the way his patients react to the infection. Dr Gibson explains:

'In a given epidemic, the same virus may attack people in different ways. There is the case where the patient feels achey, lethargic, dizzy and very weak; he just wants to go to bed and be left alone, and frequently complains of a terrible headache. For that type of individual we would use a remedy called gelsemium, which comes from yellow jasmine. In the same epidemic, another individual may have 'flu, but the symptom pattern will be quite different; this time he may have diarrhoea, vomiting, fear, anxiety, shivering, a burning heat and desire for cold water. Now in that case we would prescribe a remedy derived from arsenic because his symptoms are rather like arsenic poisoning. And yet another individual, during the same epidemic, may be struck down quite suddenly with a severe headache. He gets extremely irritable, cannot stand noises or disturbances and finds that even lifting his hand is an effort because it makes his headache worse. The only thing he wants is a cool drink and to be left to himself, preferably in a darkened room. For him the remedy is Bryonia alba . . .'

Homoeopathic medicines

Most homoeopathic remedies are derived from plants which have a long history as herbal medicines. Others are based on heavy metals, such as arsenic and gold, and others again are made from infectious

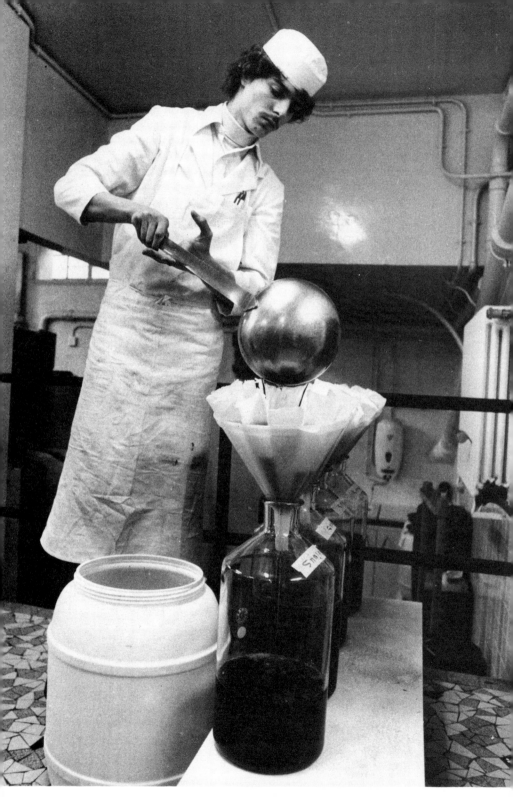

bacteria taken from the sputum of patients. There is a theoretical similarity between this last type of homoeopathic remedy and vaccination, in which a small amount of bacteria is injected into the body to encourage the immune system to produce antibodies against any future attack. However, homoeopathic remedies are prepared quite differently from vaccines and herbal medicines. The original extract is first mixed with nine or ninety-nine parts of water, lactose or alcohol and subjected to succussion, which today is generally done by machine rather than by hand. This process may then be repeated several times, taking one part of the diluted and succussed preparation and mixing it again with nine or ninety-nine parts of the solvent. Obviously, before long the amount of the original extract remaining in the mixture is very small. Indeed, some of the potencies commonly used by homoeopaths are dilutions of $1:10^{60}$, at which stage there is mathematically only a slim chance that even one molecule of the original extract still remains.

How the drugs work

Homoeopaths have been hard pressed to provide an explanation as to how infinitesimal or possibly even non-existent doses can have any effect. Some have produced theoretical explanations, which may sound rather fanciful. Some, for instance, suggest that dilution and succussion somehow separates the energy of the medicine from its material substance. Others have suggested that the pressure of succussion forces the molecules of the water or solvent into patterns around the molecules of the extract, and that these patterns remain after all material traces of the original extract have disappeared, rather like a ghost who haunts his home long after his death.

A few homoeopaths have conducted laboratory experiments to see whether homoeopathically diluted substances can have any measurable effect on plants or simple life forms, and some of them have had success. Professor Netien and his colleagues at the University of Lyons in France, for instance, found in 1970 that plants which had been poisoned with copper sulphate could be revived by feeding them a very diluted preparation of the same substance. In 1954, Professor W. E. Boyd, a Glasgow physician, published in the *British Journal of Homoeopathy* the results of a series of experiments in which he had demonstrated that homoeopathically prepared doses of mercuric chloride containing only one part in 10^{60} of the chemical

An early stage of preparing homoeopathic remedies

had a measurable effect on enzyme reactions, in this case the hydrolysis of starch by diastase. Studies like these are very interesting, and suggest that there may be some kind of energy operating at submolecular levels. But not many such experiments have been done, nor have they been published in the more widely read scientific journals, nor have they been repeated by other researchers. One of the problems faced by scientifically inclined homoeopaths is that there are few of them with time and facilities to do the kind of research which is necessary for homoeopathy to establish a sound reputation in the scientific community. Doctors at the Royal London Homoeopathic Hospital have recently embarked on a programme of research in which they are repeating experiments made by German homoeopaths which indicated that homoeopathic potencies could affect the growth of seedlings. But this research is not yet complete, and the results will not be known for some time.

Some of the lower-potency homoeopathic remedies do still contain traces of the original extract, and there is circumstantial evidence that even a few molecules could achieve a physical effect on the body. It is known, for instance, that people who are allergic to certain chemicals will react to the tiniest exposure. Industrial workers who become sensitive to platinum salts will develop a large weal on their skin if they are injected with a solution containing just a few molecules of these salts. Similarly, workers who are allergic to industrial gases suffer asthma attacks when, in laboratory conditions, they are made to breathe air containing one part in a billion of the gas.

One method of desensitising people with allergies is to give them a series of injections, beginning with one which contains the tiniest amount of the substance to which they are allergic and then gradually increasing the dose until they develop tolerance to it. However, this is not really the same as homoeopathic practice, in which the patient is given tablets containing the diluted extract to take orally.

Success of homoeopathic treatment

Sceptics maintain that any success claimed for homoeopathy must be due to a placebo response. Recently, however, Dr Robin Gibson and Dr Alistair MacNeill completed a series of clinical trials in Glasgow on patients with rheumatoid arthritis which showed that homoeopathic treatment was considerably more effective than placebo. The trials were carried out under the supervision of a university professor at the Centre for Rheumatic Diseases, which is a highly respected clinical and teaching centre. In the first trial, fifty patients with rheumatoid arthritis were given aspirin, which is still a widely used drug for this disease, whereas another fifty patients were given homoeopathic remedies. The homoeopathically treated patients were still allowed to keep on taking any conventional medicine they had been prescribed. At the end of the twelve-month study, over forty per cent of the homoeopathically treated patients had been able to give up all their conventional drugs and had improved in terms of pain and mobility. Another twenty-five per cent were physically improved, though still taking some conventional medication. The remainder did not appear to have benefited from homoeopathy in any significant way. These results were markedly better than those in the group of patients who had been given aspirin, eighty-five per cent of whom had dropped out of the study due to the side effects of the drug or its failure to relieve their pain.

The second trial was conducted 'double blind', so that neither the doctors nor the patients knew who was receiving homoeopathic treatment. The homoeopathic doctors were allotted another fifty patients with rheumatoid arthritis, all of whom were examined and treated in the same way, except that half of them were given placebo tablets instead of the actual remedy the homoeopaths had chosen for them. As in the previous trial, all the patients continued to take any conventional therapy which had been prescribed. This is admittedly a rather unusual procedure in clinical trials, but it had to be done this way because the specialists supervising Gibson and Mac-Neill's study were unwilling to see their patients abandoned to homoeopathy or placebo alone. Nevertheless, after three months the patients were examined by four independent medical assessors, and it was found that those who had been given the homoeopathic remedies had significantly improved, whereas those on placebo had tended to deteriorate. The trial was continued for another three months, but the groups were switched so that those who had previously received placebos now got homoeopathic remedies and vice versa. The patients receiving homoeopathic treatment for the first time were significantly better after three months. 'After that trial,' says Dr Gibson, 'we are quite happy to state categorically that homoeopathy is not a placebo. It is a very valuable therapeutic advance in the management of rheumatoid arthritis.'

The results of the first trial were published in the *British Journal of Clinical Pharmacology*, perhaps the last place you would expect to find homoeopathy being taken seriously. Dr Gibson and his colleagues have just finished another study, as yet unpublished, on homoeopathy and allergy, a field in which homoeopathy is claimed to be particularly effective. 'We used a technique which allows you to measure the movement of the macrophage cells which engulf foreign bodies in the blood,' Dr Gibson explains. 'We have found that these cells move quite differently in people with allergies once they have been treated with the appropriate homoeopathic remedy.'

These trials are among the first which homoeopaths in Britain have conducted, and sceptics may demand to see the results of several more before they renounce their doubts. Not all recent trials have been as successful as Dr Gibson's. Doctors at the Royal London Homoeopathic Hospital conducted a small trial of homoeopathy against placebo in the treatment of allergy which showed no significant advantage for homoeopathy. Dr Michael Jenkins, a consultant at that hospital, points out that clinical trials of homoeopathy are particularly difficult to perform because they involve many more variables than does a conventional drug trial:

'In a conventional drug trial you are simply using one drug against the disease. But with homoeopathy, where you have to match the patient with the particular remedy which suits him best as an individual, the clinical trial may involve many different prescriptions. The fact that a patient did not respond could be due to the doctor choosing the wrong remedy rather than to a failure of homoeopathy itself.'

Why choose homoeopathy?

Dr Jenkins finds that the majority of patients who come for homoeopathic treatment in his hospital have been dissatisfied in some way with conventional treatment. 'Some of them object in principle to taking what they regard as potentially dangerous drugs, and many with chronic disorders want to cut down the number of conventional drugs they have to take.'

One of the benefits of homoeopathy to emerge from Dr Gibson's trials was that no one complained of unpleasant side effects from their homoeopathic treatment. This must be an important consideration for anyone with a chronic disorder who faces a lifetime of medical treatment. Even if there is little prospect of their getting much better, they can be assured that homoeopathic treatment will not make them worse!

According to Dr John English, a London GP who is also a

homoeopath, homoeopathy also has a useful place in treating the everyday complaints. He was himself converted to homoeopathy after a colleague had successfully treated his children:

'About eighteen years ago my children got an ear infection after they had had measles. The infection was caused by a rather nasty staphylococcus called staph 80, *for which the conventional treatment at the time was a mixture of chloramphenicol and erythromycin, and chloramphenicol had a bad reputation for causing blood disorders and other problems, especially in children. So I was not keen on using them, and as a result the children had their ear infections for a long time and were also generally rather sickly. Then a friend of mine who practised homoeopathy came along and said, "Staphylococcal infection following measles, I think I can deal with that," and gave them a dose of* morbillinum, *a homoeopathic remedy derived from sputum taken from patients with measles. Their infections cleared up and slowly and gently over the next three months they returned to being the sort of children we had forgotten they ever were. I was impressed.'*

Dr English finds that acute infections respond very promptly if he selects the right remedy for the patient. 'The nice thing is that the patient often feels much better before the infection actually clears up, whereas with conventional medicine he might not feel well till after the infection had gone.' However, he would not claim that homoepathy was a cure-all or could replace allopathic medicine altogether:

'If you are treating something like advanced osteoarthritis, it would be unreasonable to expect your patient to get back the kind of joints they had when they were twenty-one. You look for reasonable relief from pain and stiffness and increased mobility, and we get that in a reasonable proportion of patients. If I was faced with a case of acute appendicitis, I could not guarantee that homoeopathy would be successful and would rush them off to an orthodox surgeon. Homoeopathy does work as well as conventional drugs for some people. For perhaps twenty-five per cent it does not seem to work at all. In others you have to combine homoeopathy with orthodox treatment to get the best results, but even then you can reduce the dose of the orthodox drug, which reduces the risk and reduces the cost, because homoeopathic remedies are much less expensive and do not have side effects.'

As with acupuncture, we find that a proportion of patients do very well on homoeopathy, although a similar proportion do not respond at all. This is also found in orthodox medicine, where even the most tried and tested drugs are seldom claimed to have a hundred-per-cent success. Obviously, a great deal depends on an accurate diagnosis, and choosing the therapy which suits the patient to a tee. Homoeopaths find that the people who respond best tend to be those who fit into one of a number of classical types. These types have been named after the remedy which suits them best. As Dr Michael Jenkins explains, the *pulsatilla* type is:

'a rather sympathetic sort, often blonde, who likes a lot of fuss made of her, needs consolation, tends to be tearful and subject to rapid changes of mood, and dislikes heat and fatty foods.'

The *sepia* type, on the other hand, tends to be:

'depressed, tired-looking, sallow. Many women become sepia *at some stage of their lives, getting fed up with the children, feeling like walking out, often with gynaecological problems as well.'*

Whatever complaint these types may present to the doctor, they will often do best on the remedy they are named after.

Although homoeopathy is one of the few alternative therapies available within the National Health Service, its practitioners are few in number and their influence is small. In 1977, orthodox consultants in Liverpool tried to prevent the city's consultant homoeopathic physician from being allocated rooms in the new teaching hospital, claiming that the presence of a homoeopathic clinic would be an undesirable influence on students and 'cause alarm to doctors and patients'. In 1980, the Camden and Islington Area Health Authority wanted to close down a large part of the Royal London Homoeopathic Hospital. Both these moves were successfully resisted, and in 1980 the Minister of Health, Dr Gerard Vaughan, repeated the assurances made by previous holders of his office that homoeopathy would be allowed to continue in the Health Service as long as there were patients wanting homoeopathic treatment and doctors available to offer it.

5 Herbalists and Hakims

Suffering from a cold? Well, take a handful of peppermint leaves, crush them and infuse them in boiling water. This peppermint tea will give symptomatic relief from a headache and runny nose. If you are troubled by a cough, rub garlic on your chest. It will not only 'loosen' your chest; it will also keep your friends and family away so that they do not catch your bug!

Herbal remedies for everyday ailments are part of our folklore. They are associated with old crones stealing out to the crossroads under the full moon to find ingredients for their magic potions and with a multitude of other whimsical superstitions. As a result, not many people with a modern scientific turn of mind feel inclined to take the subject of herbalism too seriously. It is regarded as a quaint reminder of our simple and ignorant past, when we knew little of chemistry and pharmacology. Nevertheless, herbal medicine still flourishes in this country, and in many Third World countries it is the basis of available medical care. Moreover, although the historical roots of herbalism are interwoven with astrology and magic, a great deal of the herbal medicine practised today is based on scientific principles and practical experience.

Herbalism did, of course, begin as a practical art. Leaves or moss would be used to protect wounds and sores, and our forebears would notice that some of these plants appeared to make the wound heal faster. They would also have realised that some plants had an effect on the digestive system soothing the gut in some cases and causing constipation or diarrhoea in others.

The magical, religious or astrological qualities attributed to these plants came later. Once it was realised that they had some healing power, the plants were respected and revered. As their power could not be explained in the kind of chemical terms we use today, it was assumed to be a gift from the gods or due to the presence of a spirit. In the Middle Ages, astrologers drew great significance from correlations between the time at which a plant came into flower and the position of the heavenly bodies. Alchemists, the mystical predecessors of modern research chemists, believed that dew was one of the purest substances in the universe, and therefore put great value on plants which held dew. They mistook the sticky syrup which the sundew plant secretes to attract insects as a kind of everlasting dew, and therefore came to the idea that the plant was a recipe for eternal youth. Other plants were held in awe because of their shape: much of the mystique which surrounds ginseng and mandragora, for instance, is due to the rather humanoid shape into which their roots often grow.

These associations are very poetic, but they tended to turn herbalism into more of an art than a science. Although some herbalists today see beauty and significance in the myths and legends about their raw materials, most want to establish herbalism on a more contemporary scientific footing.

One of the first and most famous attempts to separate fact from legend in herbal medicine was Dr William Withering's study of the foxglove. In 1775, this English physician was shown a herbal brew which a 'wise woman' in Shropshire was selling as a cure for dropsy. Dropsy is the oedema, or swelling, which results from the body retaining water, and it occurs most often in heart disease, when the heart is not strong enough to flush fluid from the tissues. The wise woman's brew was very effective at curing the dropsy, but it was a concotion of several herbs, any of which could have been effective ingredient. By means of trial and elimination Dr Withering ascertained that the important ingredient in the brew was root of foxglove. He subsequently made his own foxglove preparations, using various parts of the plant and trying them out on his patients. He finally discovered that the most useful part of the plant was in fact the leaf, and that it was at its most potent when the flower was in bloom. The leaf of the foxglove (or *Digitalis*, to give it its botanical Latin name) is still used by doctors today. We now know that it acts on the heart muscle, encouraging it to beat more strongly.

Medicines from plants, extracts and synthetic derivations

Several other drugs used today come directly from plants. Vinblastine and vincristine, which are used in the treatment of certain cancers, are derived from the Madagascan periwinkle. This plant had been used by traditional healers against diabetes, and chemists first began testing it as a possible source of new drugs for this disease. It was almost by chance that they found that it was more effective against tumours. The snakeroot plant, *Rauwolfia*, has been used for centuries in India as a sedative. It was not until the 1950s that an Indian medical research team investigated the chemical structure of the plant and found that its most potent ingredient was the alkaloid, reserpine. Reserpine turned out to be effective at reducing high blood pressure, though the drug has lost favour with doctors in recent years because it can have unpleasant side effects, such as depression and vertigo.

Until early this century the vast majority of medicines available to doctors were based on herbs, and many still in use today are synthetic versions of chemicals extracted from plants. The herbal ancestor of aspirin is salicin, an extract of willow bark; and a number of local anaesthetics are synthetic variations on the chemical structure of cocaine, which comes direct from the leaf of the South American coca plant. However, although the inspiration for these drugs came from herbal medicines, aspirin and novocaine today contain no plant material; they are manufactured in chemical factories where little vegetation is to be seen.

The trend of modern pharmaceutical chemistry has been to isolate the active ingredients of plant remedies and, where possible, to make a synthetic equivalent of that ingredient. The rationale for this is that pure, synthetic products are much easier to make into safe, effective medicines because you can accurately measure to the nearest milligramme how much of the chemical is being administered to the patient. Many herbalists, however, disagree with this approach, and claim that herbal medicines are safer, gentler and more acceptable to the body. Taking *Rauwolfia* as an example, they point out that no one had had problems with snakeroot until doctors gave patients its isolated alkaloid, reserpine. Taken whole in a herbal tea, they say, *Rauwolfia* would not have strong side effects. According to John Hyde, president of the National Institute of Medical Herbalists, herbal medicines have a number of built-in safeguards which are missing in synthetic drugs:

'The principal safeguard is that the natural plant contains many substances which balance each other out and thus reduce the toxic effect which can be caused by an isolated active ingredient. Take, for example, the plant Ephedra, *which is a natural source of the drug ephedrine. Ephedrine by itself has been used to control asthma, but it also makes the blood pressure*

rise, which reduces its usefulness as a drug. But if we examine the plant Ephedra we find that it contains other substances such as norephedrine and pseud-ephedrine which have a slightly antagonistic effect to ephedrine and therefore buffer its action. Thus you can relieve asthma with a remedy based on the whole plant without fear of upsetting the blood pressure. The other important safeguard is that the body is better able to cope with a natural plant in its natural state because the medicinal substances in the plant are more dilute than they would be in a synthetic medicine. The stomach can quickly reject something which is too strong for it. But natural protective mechanisms cannot cope with a synthetic drug in the same way, especially, of course, if it is injected.'

Is herbal medicine safe and effective?

In pamphlets distributed in their consulting rooms, Mr Hyde and his colleagues declare that herbal medicine is 'the safe and effective alternative' to modern drugs, a claim which we have heard made by healers, homoeopaths and acupuncturists. But how sound are these assertions in the case of herbalism?

Dr Peter Hylands, a pharmacist at Chelsea College, London, is one scientist who is generally very sympathetic towards herbal medicine, but he is not convinced by all the claims made by herbalists. There is some evidence, he says, that treatment with the whole plant, as with *Digitalis* and *Rauwolfia*, causes fewer problems than the isolated chemical ingredients. 'But in many cases I think the claim is unjustified because the scientific work necessary to validate the claim just has not been done.'

It is not reasonable to claim, Dr Hylands believes, that just because a herbal remedy is 'natural' it is necessarily safe. Plenty of plants are outright poisons, and there are others with medicinal properties which may have just as many unpleasant side effects as synthetic drugs. *Digitalis* leaf is a case in point; although it is very effective, an excessive dose can overstimulate the heart. Other well-known side effects of *Digitalis* include diarrhoea, headache and drowsiness.

There are other problems which worry him about herbal medicine practised by medically unqualified or inexperienced practitioners:

'Firstly you have to be very well trained to be able to diagnose illness correctly, and unless you can diagnose properly you are unlikely to prescribe safely. Secondly you have to know exactly what you are prescribing. A good proportion of the plant material used in herbalism is imported or of poor

quality. It is not easy to identify a sackful of dried leaves, but unless you do know what is in that sack you could be using the wrong plant!'
John Hyde answers such criticisms by pointing out that members of the Institute of Medical Herbalists all have a basic training in medicine and medical law from a four-year part-time course of study, and would prescribe permitted herbal products only within safe, legal limits.

Many of the plants which herbalists used to use freely are now restricted so that they can be prescribed only by a doctor or sold by a registered pharmacist. Herbalists who are neither doctors nor pharmacists can no longer sell preparations made from *Digitalis*, *Rauwolfia*, Canadian hemp, poison ivy, slippery elm bark, mistletoe berries, male fern and a number of other plants. Some herbal preparations may be sold by a herbalist only if the bottle or packet in which they are presented clearly states the maximum dose. Regulations introduced by the government in 1978 laid down what the maximum dose should be for potent herbs such as aconite, belladonna, cinchona, ephedra, lobelia, poison oak, ragwort and about a dozen others.

The Medicines Act of 1968 stipulated that no one could manufacture or sell a medicinal product without a licence from the government. Any new drug which comes on to the market, whether it is herbal or synthetic, must first have undergone extensive trials on animals and humans, and the Department of Health has to have been satisfied that it is efficacious and hygienically manufactured. These regulations make it hard for herbalists, who do not have the financial resources of the large pharmaceutical companies, to bring out new products. Nevertheless, the law does allow for some exemptions, which makes life easier for the herbalists. Firstly, any product which was already on the market before 1968 has a 'licence of right', which means that it can continue to be manufactured and sold. A government committee, the Committee for the Review of Medicines, is currently examining products which have a 'licence of right' and will weed out those which appear to be either unsafe or ineffective. But as there are several thousand products with a 'licence of right', it will take the committee many years to assess them all.

Herbalists are also protected by an exemption in the Medicines Act which says that they do not have to have a licence as long as the product they are selling simply consists of a plant which has been dried, crushed or chopped into small pieces before being made into pills or diluted with water. Some herbal medicines are made by steeping the plant in alcohol to draw out its chemical ingredients, but herbalists are allowed to sell products like this as long as they are manufactured on their private premises and sold only to individual patients who ask for treatment.

Like any other medically unqualified practitioner, herbalists are forbidden by law to perform abortions or even to claim that they have an effective treatment for certain diseases, which include cancer, arthritis, glaucoma, veneral disease, cataracts and diabetes. There is nothing in the law to prevent them treating people with these diseases; they are simply not allowed to say that they can treat them. This can put the herbalist in a strange position, as John Hyde pointed out:

'It is well known that a number of herbs can lower blood sugar and therefore be useful against diabetes. One of these is goat's rue, Galliga officinalis, another is Eugenia jambolana, and there are others mentioned in the pharmacology textbooks. But if someone comes to me and asks me whether I can help their diabetes, I cannot tell them that I can. All I can say is that I can offer them something to help their general health.'

Plant resources

There are about 300,000 plants in the world which have been named and classified so far. It is quite possible that many of them will be useful as medicines or foodstuffs, but as yet only a tiny proportion of them have been even cursorily investigated for possible medicinal properties. In Britain, there are several hundred specimens in the herbarium at Kew Gardens which have been brought by botanists from the four corners of the globe and which are reputed, according to local information gathered by the botanists, to have healing properties of one kind or another. Dr Peter Hylands was one of a group of scientists who recently launched an appeal for funds to have these plants investigated further:

'Many plant drugs have entered modern medicine as a result of someone following up the folklore attached to them. Much of this folklore information has been recorded at places like Kew, and it would not be very difficult to take the plants which have some reputed pharmacological action and test them in a laboratory. This would certainly take time and money, but we should remember that about half the prescriptions filled today are for substances which are closely related chemically to substances found in the plant kingdom.'

In 1970, the Swiss herbal medicine company Bio-Strath AG financed a research programme on herbal medicines which was carried out by scientists at North East London Polytechnic. The London naturopath Michael van Straten, who helped to organise this research, relates that the project yielded many interesting and surprising results:

'We found that a lot of herbs which have been traditionally used for medicinal purposes had no apparent pharmacological action at all. Others did not have the action they were reputed to have, and we found others again which had very potent effects, even though they were not listed in the old pharmacopoeias. Juniper oil, which is listed in the herbal literature as a diuretic (i.e. it makes you pass water) showed no such activity in our laboratory tests. We found from animal experiments that Passion Flower leaves, Passiflora incarnata, *acted on the heart rather like* Digitalis, *though it was less potent. A combination of extracts of Passion Flower, hawthorn and arnica was found to be extremely valuable pharmacologically as a heart stimulant, though milder and potentially less toxic than* Digitalis. *We found that extract of primula root was extremely effective at reducing arthritic inflammation in animals, and did not have the gastric side effects which often occur with aspirin. We found that bearberry leaves,* Uvae ursi, *were an extremely powerful natural antibiotic which could be useful in the treatment of skin conditions. In our laboratory trials bearberry prevented the growth of six common bacterial organisms, including* E. coli *and* Staph. aureus.'*

Herbal medicine is not being entirely neglected by the official medical agencies. The World Health Organisation has made the investigation and development of traditional medicine part of its policy. It has set up a research institute in Rome where scientists will study the pharmacological activity of plant remedies from Third World countries. It has also sponsored a research project to investigate the herbal treatment used in traditional Ayurvedic medicine in India against rheumatoid arthritis. Dr Hylands suggests that the poorer countries of the Third World, which do not have a developed pharmaceutical industry, stand to benefit most from investment in herbal medicine. He points out, for example, that oleander, which is a common plant in East Africa, is known to contain a useful heart stimulant. Given good production facilities, East African countries could manufacture a medicine from oleander which would save them from having to import digitalis and other drugs from Europe and America.

However, there are two problems which may prevent such countries from exploiting their natural plant resources. Firstly, many doctors and pharmacists who are trained in the West lose interest in the traditional forms of medicine used in their countries, and want to practise the Western-style medicine they have been taught. Secondly, Third World governments have grown wary of being exploited by foreign entrepreneurs. As Dr Hylands explains, 'They believe that if they let foreigners with money in to develop the resource, it will be the foreigners who enjoy the profit. They fear that if they let their valuable plant material out of the country, it will not come back to them.'

Hakims

In this context, it is ironic that one of the most popular forms of herbal medicine being practised in Britain today has itself been imported from the Third World. Due to the growth of the Asian immigrant population, there are now almost as many *hakims* offering traditional Asian therapies as there are native British herbalists.

Hakim means 'wise man', and it is the title given to practitioners of the Unani system of medicine practised in the Muslim areas of India and Pakistan. Its historical roots lie in the ancient Greek medicine established by Hippocrates and his colleagues on the island of Cos around 400 BC and in the Arabic medical tradition founded by Avicenna (Ibn Sina) about a thousand years ago. In practice, however, it has a great deal in common with the Ayurvedic medical system which is part of the Hindu Indian tradition. Ayurvedic practitioners are called *veyds*, but in the past few centuries *hakims* and *veyds* have borrowed much from each other's ideas and practices. Most of the traditional Asian practitioners at work in Britain are Muslims and basically follow Unani principles, so for the sake of simplicity I shall refer to them all as *hakims*.

Like the traditional Chinese physician, the *hakim* attaches great significance to the pulse when making a diagnosis. He seeks many qualities in it which are unknown to the Western doctor but which give him important information about the balance of elements and energies in the patient's mind and body. *Hakims* also classify their patients' condition and the medicines they prescribe according to a system of 'humours'. The theory of humours is not easy to translate into contemporary Western terminology, though it has strong similarities with a medical and philosophical theory which was developed in Greece in the fifth century BC and which was followed in Europe well into the period of the Renaissance.

The humours are based on the philosopher Empedocles' theory that all matter was based on four elements: fire, air, earth and water. Fire was hot and dry, air was hot and wet, earth was cold and dry, and water was cold and wet. The body contained four vital fluids corresponding to these elements. 'Yellow bile' corresponded to fire, blood to air, 'black bile' to earth, and phlegm to water.

The balance of these vital fluids or humours controlled the individual's health and temperament. Someone in whom the hot, dry yellow bile was the dominant humour would be *choleric* and prone to fits of anger. The *sanguine* temperament was due to a dominance of blood, and the *melancholy* temperament was due to an excess of black bile. The dominant humour in the *phlegmatic* personality was, of course, phlegm. The various treatments used by mediaeval physicians, such as blood letting, purges and emetics, were supposed to release harmful excesses of a particular humoral fluid.

The *hakim* approaches his patient rather like the mediaeval European physician. The four qualities he looks for are *saffra* (hot and dry), *khun** (hot and wet), *soda* (cold and dry) and *balram* (cold and wet). These qualities can allegedly be detected from the pulse and also from the patient's physical appearance and symptoms. A *balram* type would be overweight and sweaty, whereas a *saffra* type would be lean and underweight. A patient who said that he had a sweet, phlegmy taste in his mouth would probably have an excess of *balram*, and someone who complained of a hot, salty dryness in his mouth would have too much *saffra*. Nose bleeds might be due to too much *khun**, and a shivery chill could be attributed to *soda*.

The remedies used by the *hakim* are also classified according to their heat, dryness, coldness or wetness, and the correct prescription is one which counteracts the patient's own condition. The herb turmeric, for instance, is thought to be hot and dry and is therefore used in the treatment of diabetes, which is generally classified as a cold, wet *balram* condition.

These principles are even used in Asian cooking. A West London *hakim*, A. Q. Salimi, suggested to me that a lot of Britons who get stomach troubles after eating curry would suffer less if they made sure that the hot, dry chili in their curry powder was balanced with cold, wet coriander! Hakim Salimi points out that the heat or dryness of a person or food does not necessarily correspond to any physically measurable quality. It more concerns taste and feeling.

*The *kh* is pronounced as a guttural *h*, as in Khomeini.

Hakim Salimi learned his trade from his father, who had learnt it from his father before him. In Pakistan, where traditional Unani medicine is still the backbone of the health service, *hakims* are trained either by apprenticeship or at Unani medical colleges which run four-year degree courses. *Hakims* have recently been able to obtain licences, and the college graduates are classified Grade A *hakims*, whereas those like Hakim Salimi who learned their skills as apprentices are Grade B. Unfortunately, not all the practitioners in this country who call themselves *hakims* have had any formal training. Some are entrepreneurs or plain quacks, who have noticed a demand from the Asian immigrant community for traditional medicine and have exploited it. Hakim Salimi is an exception in another way: whereas most *hakims* draw their patients from the Asian community, many of those who come to his London practice are native English people who prefer 'natural' medicine to conventional medical therapies.

Hakims in Britain

The first occasion on which *hakims* came to official notice in Britain was in 1976, when the Department of Health received a letter from Mohammed Aslam, a pharmacist then working at the University of Aston. Aslam had been making a study of the way in which patients took drugs they had been prescribed, whether they followed or, indeed, always understood the directions given to them by their doctors. (It has been estimated that at least a third of the medicines prescribed on the National Health Service are wasted because people either take them wrongly or do not take them at all!) His investigations took him into the homes of many Asian immigrant families, where he found that a lot of patients were taking a variety of exotic medicines which had certainly not been obtained from an NHS doctor or chemist. When he asked where the medicines had come from, he was told time and again that they had been prescribed 'by the *hakim*'. 'I wrote to the Department of Health asking them to tell me what they knew about *hakims*. I got a letter back asking, "What is a *hakim*?" '

Finding the answer to this question became the subject of Mohammed Aslam's PhD thesis, which he completed at Nottingham University with the help of a grant from the Department of Health. He found that there are three kinds of *hakim* practising in Britain: resident *hakims* who have learnt their trade in India or Pakistan and who practise in this country full-time; visiting *hakims*, who tend to be well known in the sub-continent and who fly to Britain occasionally after advertising their services in Asian language newspapers; and part-time *hakims*, most of whom are untrained and sell imported medicines as a profitable sideline or to help out friends and family.

Aslam concluded that generally speaking, *hakims* were performing a useful service to their patients. The majority of patients he questioned were well satisfied with the treatment that they had been receiving even though it was sometimes expensive. (Visiting *hakims* often charge fees on a sliding scale, ranging from around £20 for 'basic treatment' to £200 for 'excellent treatment'.) *Hakims* could often communicate with Asian patients who spoke poor English much better than their GP could. They also had a very good understanding of their patient's social and cultural background, thus giving them an insight into many psychological and psychosexual problems, which accounted for a large proportion of the complaints brought to them.

Some remedies used by hakims

However, there were some aspects of the *hakims'* work which caused Aslam concern. Some of the medicines and tonics they prescribed contained potentially toxic heavy metals, such as lead, arsenic and gold. Most of the herbal remedies were completely unknown in this country, were unlicensed, and their pharmacological action, if any, was a mystery. Some of the herbs they used were undeniably effective, but could present problems for the patient if they were taken at the same time as drugs prescribed by a doctor. Also there were instances where patients who were quite severely ill had been given useless medicines by a *hakim* when they would have been better off with conventional Western medicine.

Heavy metals are used predominantly in two kinds of preparation used in Asian medicine. Firstly, there are the *kushtay*, tonics which are most commonly sold as cures for impotence, premature ejaculation and other sexual disorders, or quite simply as aphrodisiacs to individuals who want to improve their sexual performance. *Kushtay* means 'conquered' or 'killed', and it is a term applied to all medicinal products which have been burnt and rendered to ash. Arsenic, for instance, would be made into *kushtay* by heating it so that it oxidised. Shells, herbs and pearls also go into *kushtay*. *Kushtay* made from egg-shells or oyster shells are given for bladder problems, and burnt pearls are used for treating certain heart conditions. Heavy metals have been used in Ayurvedic medicine for centuries without widespread alarm about their toxicity, though this could be because no one has thought to look out for long-term toxic effects of mild amounts of poison. Dr Aslam points out that the methods for making *kushtay* may be better in Asia:

'Not all the oxides of arsenic are poisonous. Arsenic pentoxide is harmless and occurs in salt and seafood. Arsenic trioxide can kill you. In India and Pakistan the manufacturers of kushtay *know how to control the oxidisation process so they know how to get the pentoxide, but the* hakims *here have poorer facilities. I have found people trying to make* kushtay *on their kitchen stove.'*

Heavy metals are also used in *surma,* a cosmetic which is applied to the eyes of women and children as an 'eye brightener' and to ward off the Evil Eye. *Surma* is a traditional product, and the Prophet Muhammad is said to have recommended its use. Aslam and his colleagues at Nottingham University have found that Asian children in Bradford tend to have higher levels than normal of lead in their blood, and he has attributed this to the use of *surma* containing lead sulphide.

In 1978, the Department of Health, acting on Dr Aslam's advice, banned a medicine called Bal Jivan Chamcho which was being imported from India as a tonic for babies. The tonic consisted of a lump of herbal material contained in a metal spoon. It was not the herbs which worried Aslam; it was the spoon, which was made of lead. The tonic was prepared by pouring hot water on to the lump of herbal material in the spoon; the liquid infusion, which was bound to have picked up lead in the process, was then given to the baby.

The use of lead in *hakims'* medicines attracted considerable publicity in 1979, much to the annoyance of many *hakims.* Hakim Salimi and Hakim Dharampal, secretary of the recently formed Association of Unani and Ayurvedic Practitioners in the United Kingdom, both assured me that poisonous heavy metals were not used in their medicines nor in any traditional Unani preparation. They pointed out that most brands of *surma* are based on zinc or antimony rather than lead, and are therefore not dangerous. On the other hand, I met a *hakim* in Yorkshire who declared that concern about lead was a silly nonsense trumped up by 'ignorant' Western science, and that although lead might be toxic to Europeans it was not toxic when given to Asians in a medicine prepared by a *hakim*! He probably represents an extreme point of view, however.

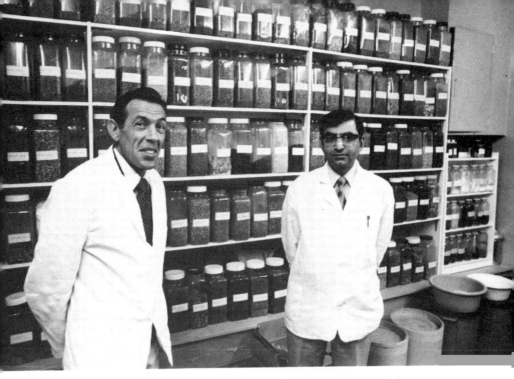

East meets West: an English herbalist and a hakim in their London clinic

Some of the herbal medicines that Dr Aslam has collected are undeniably useful. The liquorice root, *Glycyrrhiza*, for example, has been used in the East and the West for centuries, and has proven value in relieving inflammation of the bronchial and intestinal tracts. There are others which might, given more intensive research, prove useful to the West.

Two of these are *Abrus precatorius* and *Andrographis paniculata*. The seeds of *Abrus* are about an eighth of an inch in diameter and striped red and black. The seed is poisonous if chewed, but if its husk is removed and the inner part is rolled and made into tablets which are swallowed (the stomach acid neutralises any remaining poison), it appears to be an effective contraceptive for women. Dr Aslam warns that no proper studies have been done to test whether *Abrus* has any long-term toxic effects or whether it can affect the foetus in subsequent pregnancies. However, he has seen it used by *hakims* in hospitals in Delhi, and spoken with their female patients who agreed that it was an effective contraceptive. It is sold as a contraceptive by some *hakims* in Britain. *Andrographis* does not seem to be used here, though it has acquired a reputation in the East as an effective contraceptive for men. Animal tests have been performed in India which showed that it did significantly reduce the sperm count and that the sperm appeared to return to normal after the herb was taken out of the animals' diet.

Though *hakims* import some of their herbs and patent medicines, most of their raw materials would be familiar to a British herbalist or even to a keen cook. Turmeric, cardamon, thyme, pepper, garlic, mint are all old friends, though they would go through various stages of preparation before being administered to a patient. Hakim Salami, who stocks five hundred herbs, claims that a good *hakim* could tackle most problems which came his way with about a dozen:

'A hakim does not need hundreds of herbs. For example, in an emergency you can relieve the pain of toothache by rubbing half-burnt tobacco on the gum. The tobacco has a high concentration of nicotine, which will work as a local anaesthetic. If someone is suffering from a cold, you can take an onion, put it in the oven for a few minutes, then crush it and put a few drops of the juice in the nostrils. The same half-baked onion can be crushed and mixed with sodium bicarbonate to treat stomach ache. We use honey to relieve constipation and make a very fine powder of salt, which is taken as snuff to relieve headaches.'

Some of the patent medicines imported from India may look very exotic to a British customs inspector or Department of Health official, but are well known over-the-counter remedies in Asia, which have been used without any apparent untoward effect for years. There are, unfortunately, others which undoubtedly cannot live up to the claims made for them. In 1978, an Asian herbalist in Birmingham was prosecuted by the Department of Health for selling a product called Magsol. He claimed that it was an aphrodisiac, and the word was spread that it could cure venereal disease. In fact, although it cost £15 a bottle, it was made of sand and sugar.

On the other hand, the very effectiveness of some *hakims'* medicines presents a hazard if the patient is also taking drugs prescribed by the general practitioner. Dr Aslam reported a case in *The Lancet* in which a woman who was being treated for diabetes by her doctor also took a herb called Karella, which reduced blood-sugar levels. Taken together, the drug and the herb brought her blood sugar down so low that the woman came to the verge of coma. Karella is also a popular ingredient in curries, so in this case the danger is not just restricted to diabetics who seek two kinds of treatment.

This kind of problem could be overcome if *hakims* were to learn about conventional medical treatment, and if doctors were to become aware of the possibility that their patients might be consulting someone else. There are still great differences between Asian and European ideas on health, however. Western medicines are generally regarded as 'hot' by *hakims*, and a patient who was traditionally diagnosed as suffering from a 'hot' condition is likely to be advised to give up any 'hot' medicines prescribed by the GP as they could only, in the *hakim*'s opinion, make the condition worse. Similarly, pregnancy is traditionally regarded as a 'hot' condition, and Asian women are often advised – by their families as well as by *hakims* – to stop eating 'hot' foods when they are pregnant. The 'hot' foods include many of those which are rich in protein. So here traditional advice runs against Western ideas on nutrition, which suggest that protein is very necessary during pregnancy. Iron tablets, which are routinely handed out by the National Health Service to pregnant women to prevent anaemia, are also thought to be 'hot' and therefore undesirable.

Traditional ideas die hard, and there are plenty of sound moral, social and political arguments against trying to impose Western standards on an Asian community which prefers to follow its own cultural habits and beliefs. For the Department of Health, the *hakims* have proved to be a much hotter political potato than other alternative practitioners. Although it has prosecuted the manufacturer of Magsol and banned the import of the Bal Jivan Chamcho baby tonic, its attitude at present is conciliatory rather than hostile. A Department official whom we interviewed explained as follows:

'We have considered whether we should conduct some kind of purge and have decided against it, for what seem to be good tactical reasons. The hakims, *like anyone else, have the right under English common law to offer forms of treatment which are not illegal. It seems to us that if we could get alongside the* hakims *and enlist their support rather than risk driving the whole business underground, then we would stand more chance of success. While we have to follow up any infringement of the law which comes to our notice, what we would like to do in the immediate future is get in touch with local communities and enlist the support of their leaders in adopting a more enlightened approach.'*

6 Osteopathy and Chiropractic

Not many years ago osteopathy and chiropractic would have headed anyone's list of alternative therapies. These manipulative techniques were the first unconventional therapies to become popular and well organised. Although healers and herbalists had been practising in Britain for centuries, the osteopaths were the first to publicise their doctrines, establish training schools and set themselves up as a professional alternative to orthodox medicine – and succeeded in attracting the fury and contempt of the medical profession in the process.

Today, the osteopaths and chiropractors look orthodox when compared with some of the other alternatives we have seen. They do not profess exotic philosophies nor speak of energies unknown to conventional science. Their approach to the body and its disorders is basically mechanistic. The principle reason they are still regarded as unorthodox is that manipulation is still not a subject on the syllabus of medical schools.

Back pain

The spine is literally the backbone of manipulative medicine. Pains in the neck and back are the staple fare of osteopaths and chiropractors, although they do treat other complaints. Just how successful manipulators are with these disorders is hard to define with any exactness, because few large-scale clinical trials have been performed. In 1979, the government-appointed Working Group on Low Back Pain recommended that such trials needed to be conducted promptly so that everyone involved might have a clearer idea of the value and limitations of manipulation, and one study has now begun at a London teaching hospital. In the meantime, patients, who tend to rely more on personal recommendations than the results of clinical trials published in medical journals, continue to flock to the manipulators. Most of them go because they have not been able to get relief from their pain from their doctor. Many get better, but a minority have severe problems which cannot be cured by manipulation and have to return to orthodox medicine for orthopaedic surgery.

Back pain is one of the biggest medical problems today. According to the International Society for the Study of the Lumbar Spine, eighty per cent of the world's population are temporarily disabled by back-ache at some time during their life. The economic cost to Britain was recently estimated as £1 million a day, with drugs, medical treatment and sickness benefits for back injuries costing over £100 million a year and more than £200 million a year being lost to industry because of workers having to take time off. These figures take no account of personal suffering, nor of the distress and hardship caused to families when a father, mother or child is laid up with back pain.

Success rate of surgery

Orthopaedic surgery can help relieve the most serious kinds of back injury. The main operation which is performed is the laminectomy, where a layer of bone in a vertebra is removed, thus relieving pressure on the spinal cord, and surgical removal of a damaged intervertebral disc. The discs are tough, fibrous shock absorbers between the vertebrae, which can burst if subjected to prolonged or heavy pressure. When the disc bursts, jelly-like material from its interior bulges out, and can press on nerves or nerve roots, causing jabs of pain in the back or the shooting pains of sciatica. Again, once the pressure is removed, the pain should go.

Unfortunately, surgery is not always successful. The government's Working Group found that as many as one patient in three suffered back pain again after having an operation, and that one in ten had to have further surgery. Statistics collected by doctors belonging to the International Society for the Study of the Lumbar Spine suggest that the more times a patient is operated on for back pain, the lower are his chances of permanent relief.

Causes of back pain

Surgical methods may, of course, improve, but one of the main problems facing doctors and manipulators is to know exactly what the cause of a back pain is. Some disorders are very difficult to diagnose precisely. X-rays will show up fractures and misalignments of the vertebrae, and opaque substances can be injected into the spinal canal which will reveal obstructions in the canal when it is X-rayed. But the lesions which cause pain are often in nerves and soft tissues, which do not show up on X-rays.

Fortunately, the majority of back pains seem to clear up of their own accord if the injury is not severe. Simple bed-rest has been shown to be as effective as analgesic drugs in getting people back to work in cases of what is described medically as 'non-specific back pain'. This term covers the various aches, sprains and strains for which doctors cannot find a precise diagnosis. These non-specific pains account for a large proportion of the cases treated by osteopaths and chiropractors, so it is quite possible that much of the success which has been attributed to manipulation by satisfied patients is in fact due to the healing influence of nature alone.

Manipulation

One recent clinical trial did suggest that manipulation might help nature in its task. The trial involved physiotherapists at a Manchester hospital who used a technique called 'Maitland's mobilisation', and the results showed that patients who were 'mobilised' lost their pain sooner than those who were not. In the long term, however, mobilisation did not seem to reduce the chances of another attack of back pain. Osteopaths and chiropractors have pointed out that their techniques are rather different from Maitland's mobilisation, but there are still no controlled clinical trial reports to show that their methods are any more effective.

Today, no responsible practitioner would claim that he had 'the answer' to back pain. Doctors and the non-medical manipulators appear to be overcoming their old antagonism and trying to learn from each other. The government's Working Party on Low Back Pain included both kinds of practitioner, and the osteopaths' and chiropractors' professional bodies report that GPs are much more willing to refer patients to them for manipulative treatment than they used to be.

The main reason doctors used to mistrust manipulators was that they made extraordinarily bold claims about the effectiveness of manipulation. The founder of osteopathy, Andrew Taylor Still, vehemently loathed orthodox medicine and wanted to make osteopathy a complete alternative system of medicine. Serious claims were made that osteopathy or chiropractic could even cure complaints like head lice and diabetes. At the turn of the century, when the manipulative therapies were establishing themselves, there was also much more spinal tuberculosis in America and Europe than is seen today. Manipulation can make this condition very much worse, and occasionally did so.

Qualified osteopaths and chiropractors are less likely to make that kind of mistake today, as they are trained in medical diagnosis and radiography, and many actually have their own X-ray equipment. Their training courses last for four years, and the colleges employ professors and lecturers from teaching hospitals as well as experienced practitioners of the manipulative therapies. Dr John Ebbetts, former president of the British Association of Manipulative Medicine (BAMM), an organisation which trains doctors to manipulate, even believes that a trained osteopath or chiropractor can diagnose and treat musculo-skeletal disorders 'with at least as much skill as a doctor'. The advantage of good osteopathic and chiropractic training, he told me, was that the students receive many hours of practical experience under supervision, 'something which we on the medical side of the fence are unable to give our students'.

BAMM was set up by doctors who had learnt manipulation after graduating from medical school, and who believed that more of their colleagues should be taught it. It now has about three hundred members, most of whom received their manipulative training from a series of week-end courses which the association runs annually. There are three osteopathic colleges (listed in the back of this book) and a chiropractic college. There are about 750 qualified osteopaths and chiropractors practising in this country.

If patients are at risk of being misdiagnosed or mishandled by manipulators, that risk is perhaps more likely to come from the unqualified manipulators, who abound in numbers equal to those who are qualified. Anyone can call himself or herself an osteopath and put up a brass plate. The unqualified can also advertise, unlike the qualified manipulators, who are forbidden to do so by their professional bodies.

The medical manipulators – those, that is, who belong to BAMM – confine their manipulation to disorders of the spine and joints. Back and joint pain are the largest part of the osteopaths' and chiropractors' work-load too, though they do claim success with certain types of migraine, asthma, intestinal disorders and bronchial complaints. According to Audrey Smith, head of the teaching faculty at the British School of Osteopathy in London, osteopathy 'interests itself

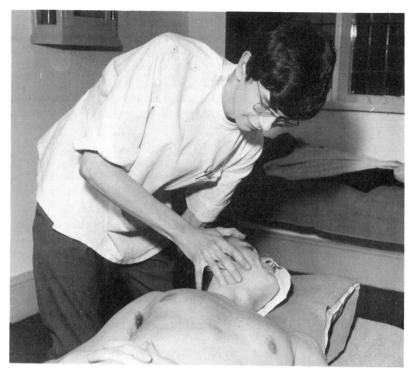

Osteopathic manipulation of the neck

chiefly in structural defects within the body, and bases its treatment principally on the musculo-skeletal system'.

What this means in practice is that osteopaths may attempt to correct any disorder which looks as if it could be put right by manual therapy. Migraine is a disease which has several possible causes, but a quite common cause, according to the manipulators, is a derangement of the cervical joints in the neck. If this is the cause, it may well be cured by manipulation. Asthma and bronchial complaints can sometimes be relieved, if not necessarily totally cured, by improving the movement of the ribs by manipulating the dorsal spine and the muscles attached to it. This allows the patient to breathe more easily. Although a responsible manipulator would not try to 'cure' a joint which was damaged by a bone infection or tumour, manipulation can relieve pain and muscle tension in the area and provide palliative relief.

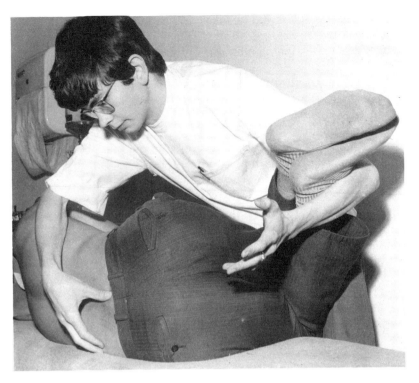

Osteopathic treatment for low back pain

Manipulative procedures range from vigorous pressure directed at a joint to gentle massage. Manipulators who are not doctors are not allowed to prescribe drugs, but some give their patients homoeopathic remedies, vitamins or dietary advice if these appear to be necessary.

Osteopath or chiropractor?

Osteopathic and chiropractic techniques overlap considerably, and a few years ago one well-known manipulator developed a therapy which he called 'osteopractic'. The main difference between the two is that osteopathy tends to use leverage, while the chiropractor goes in for more direct thrusts at the joint in question. If we take the lower part of the back, the lumbar spine, as an example, the osteopath would manipulate it by twisting the patient on his side so that the pelvis came forwards and the shoulders were thrust backwards. The shoulders and pelvis would be rotated in opposite directions until there was tension in all the spinal joints except the one which was to be manipulated. From this point a slight further rotation would move the vertebra and probably produce an audible click. A chiropractor might attempt the same task with the patient lying prone and by exerting pressure on the vertebra with the side of his hand.

Another manipulative style for disc problems has been developed by a doctor, James Cyriax, which combines manipulation with traction. Traction means pulling, and the idea is to stretch the spine, thus temporarily relieving the pressure on the intervertebral discs. A dislodged disc can then, according to Dr Cyriax, be easily manoeuvred back into its correct position. Alternatively, if the disc is ruptured and its jelly is oozing out, the release of pressure brought about by traction will cause the jelly to be sucked back inside. For injuries which will not respond to manipulation, treatment may include spinal injections of anti-inflammatory steroids and/or local anaesthetic. Unlike osteopathy and chiropractic, some of Dr Cyriax's manoeuvres require the assistance of another person, usually a physiotherapist.

7 A Consumer's Guide

Alternative medical therapies are not practised by many doctors working in the National Health Service. There are a few doctors who practise manipulation, acupuncture, hypnosis and relaxation therapies and a few rare individuals who try their hand at more unusual alternatives. GPs tend to take more practical interest in alternatives than hospital doctors, but they are unlikely to be able to practise their therapy full time in the context of a busy family practice which has to cater for all kinds of ailment. National Health Service hospitals, in so far as they allow alternative therapies to be practised on the premises at all, usually rely on the services of an individual doctor, who may attend only one half day clinic a week. Healers who are affiliated to the National Federation of Spiritual Healers are allowed by the Department of Health to minister to patients in hospital if they have been invited personally by the patient. Apart from these exceptions, alternative medicine at the present time is something which the patient has to pay for out of his own pocket.

One or two organisations like the Healing Research Trust and the newly formed Action for Natural Therapies are campaigning for the alternatives to be made available on the National Health Service, but at present it seems that the *status quo* is not likely to change in the foreseeable future. Although many alternative practitioners would like to work in the health service, the only way for them to gain admittance – unless, of course, they are doctors – is by applying as a group to be recognised as a 'profession supplementary to medicine' with similar status to physiotherapists or dieticians. Not many would be prepared to accept this status if it meant (as it almost certainly would) that diagnosis and choice of treatment remained in doctors' hands.

So where is the patient to turn? It would be difficult enough recommending ways in which readers could find a good GP or medical specialist. The professional rules of the medical profession prohibit doctors from advertising their services, and patients take pot luck either by consulting the nearest doctor at hand or by following the advice of friends and neighbours. Without friendly and informed advice, finding a competent and qualified alternative practitioner can be even more difficult. A bewildering variety of qualifications and numerous letters after the name are sported by alternative practitioners, some awarded for real academic and practical achievements, and others worth little more than the tatty document presented at the end of some postal tuition courses. Nor do qualifications necessarily mean a great deal in alternative medicine. Many reputedly good healers have no qualifications whatsoever, and there are plenty of unschooled practitioners of all sorts who have hosts of satisfied patients. The following guidance is intended for those who have no other resource than the Yellow Pages or small ads in the local press. I list the main organisations representing alternative practitioners together with the qualifications, if any, which they award.

Fees charged by practitioners vary enormously. Some healers charge nothing, others accept only donations. Most alternative practitioners, however, are in private practice and have a scale of fees, ranging from £5 to £50 or more per consultation. Be bold; don't be afraid to ask the cost *before* treatment begins! VAT at the going rate has to be charged by practitioners who are not medically qualified. Doctors do not have to charge VAT however unorthodox their therapy may be.

Orthodox medicine

Let us first look at the most common medical qualifications held by doctors:

MB, BS	*Medicinae Baccalaureus* (Bachelor of Medicine), Bachelor of Surgery
BM, BCh	Bachelor of Medicine, Bachelor of Surgery
MRCS	Member of the Royal College of Surgeons,
LRCP	Licentiate of the Royal College of Physicians
LMSSA	Licentiate in Medicine and Surgery, Society of Apothecaries

The above are all basic medical qualifications which show that the doctor has passed the examinations of his university medical school or of one of the approved examination boards.

MD   *Medicinae Doctor* (Doctor of Medicine)

All American doctors are MDs, but in Britain this degree is an added distinction, showing that the doctor has completed original research.

DO   Diploma in Ophthalmology
DCH   Diploma in Child Health
DPM   Diploma in Psychological Medicine
DA   Diploma in Anaesthetics
DRCOG   Diploma in Obstetrics and Gynaecology

The diplomas above indicate that the doctor has studied the particular speciality, though not necessarily to the standard which would get him a job as a hospital consultant.

FRCS   Fellow of the Royal College of Surgeons;
          a necessary qualification for surgeons,
          not to be confused with MRCS above
MRCP   Member of the Royal College of Physicians –
          a higher qualification, held by almost all
          consultant physicians
MRCPsych Member of the Royal College of Psychiatrists
FFARCS   Fellow of the Faculty of Anaesthetists,
          Royal College of Surgeons
MRCOG   Member of the Royal College of Obstetricians and
          Gynaecologists
FFHom   Fellow of the Faculty of Homoeopathy
MRCGP   Member of the Royal College of General Practitioners

The above qualifications indicate experience and expertise in the speciality.

Fellowship of one of the Royal Colleges (e.g. FRCP, FRCPsych, FRCOG or FRCGP) apart from the Royal College of Surgeons, is by election rather than by examination, and suggests that the doctor is very well respected by his colleagues.

| FRSM | Fellow of the Royal Society of Medicine |
| FRSH | Fellow of the Royal Society of Health |

Do not be falsely impressed by the two titles above, which do not signify academic attainment. They are available to anyone who pays the subscription to the society in question.

MSc	Master of Science
DSc	Doctor of Science
PhD	Doctor of Philosophy
DPhil	Doctor of Philosophy

The four university degrees above are awarded for research work, but they are not medical qualifications.

Acupuncture

There are three colleges which run two- or three-year part-time courses for would-be acupuncturists:

The British Acupuncture Association and Register,
34 Alderney Street, London SW1
(Tel: 01-834 1012)

Qualifications

| MBAcA | Member of the British Acupuncture Association |
| FBAcA | Fellow of the British Acupuncture Association |

The College of Traditional Chinese Acupuncture,
Queensway, Leamington Spa, Warwickshire
(Tel: 0926–22121)

Qualifications

| LicAc | Licentiate of Acupuncture |
| BAc | Bachelor of Acupuncture |

The International College of Oriental Medicine,
Green Hedges Lane, East Grinstead, Sussex
(Tel: 0342–28567)

Qualifications

| BAc | Bachelor of Acupuncture |
| DAc | Doctor of Acupuncture |

Some medically qualified doctors have learnt their acupuncture at one of these schools, while others have learnt it abroad or from short courses organised by experienced medical acupuncturists. Some medically unqualified acupuncturists style themselves 'Doctor'.

Autogenic training and Biofeedback

There are no organisations which offer qualifications in these therapies, though short courses are available at:

> The Centre for Autogenic Training,
> 12 Milford House, 7 Queen Anne Street, London W1
> (Tel: 01–637 1586)

> The Psycho-Biology Institute,
> c/o 26 Wendell Road, London W12
> (Tel: 01–743 1518)

Chiropractic

A four-year full-time training course is run at:

> Anglo-European College of Chiropractic,
> 2 Cavendish Road, Bournemouth, Dorset
> (Tel: 0202–24777)
>
> *Qualification*
DC   Doctor of Chiropractic

A list of qualified chiropractors can be obtained from:

> The British Chiropractors' Association,
> 5 First Avenue, Chelmsford, Essex
> (Tel: 0245–353078)

Hakims

This association was formed in 1980, and is compiling a register of *hakims* who qualified either in India or Pakistan or who have had apprenticeship training and practical experience:

> The Association of Unani and
> Ayurvedic Practitioners in UK,
> 12 Little Newport Street, London W1
> (Tel: 01–437 2600)

Healing

Some of the larger healers' associations which teach and keep a directory of practising healers are:

The National Federation of Spiritual Healers,
Old Manor Farm Studio, Sunbury on Thames,
Middlesex (Tel: Sunbury 83164)

The White Eagle Lodge,
New Lands, Rake, Liss, Hampshire
(Tel: 073082–3300)

Guild of Spiritualist Healers,
99 Bloomfield Road, Gloucester (Tel: 0452–25455)

Herbalism

This institute keeps a list of graduates of its four-year part-time training courses:

National Institute of Medical Herbalists,
65 Frant Road, Tunbridge Wells, Kent
(Tel: 0892–27439)

Qualification

MNIMH   Member of the National Institute of Medical Herbalists

Homoeopathy

Courses are run for doctors, and a register of homoepathic doctors is kept at:

The Faculty of Homoeopathy,
Royal London Homoeopathic Hospital,
Great Ormond Street, London WC1
(Tel: 01–837 7821)

The following society has an affiliated college which runs part-time training courses for those who are not medically qualified, and keeps a register of members:

The Society of Homoeopaths,
59 Norfolk House Road, London SW16
(Tel: 01–677 3260)

Naturopathy

This college runs a four-year full-time training course:

The British College of Naturopathy and Osteopathy,
Fraser House, 6 Netherhall Gardens, London NW3
(Tel: 01–435 8728)

Qualifications
ND   Naturopathic Diploma
DO   Diploma in Osteopathy

Graduates join the British Naturopathic and Osteopathic Association (at the same address), which keeps a register of members who may style themselves:

MBNOA   Member of the British Naturopathic and Osteopathic Association

Osteopathy

Doctors usually train at:

London College of Osteopathy,
8 Boston Place, London NW2
(Tel: 01–262 1128)

Qualification
LLCO   Licentiate of the London College of Osteopathy

A four-year full-time course is run by:

The British School of Osteopathy,
16 Buckingham Gate, London SW1
(Tel: 01–828 9479

Qualifications
DO   Diploma in Osteopathy
MRO   Member of the Register of Osteopaths

A register of osteopaths who have taken the above course is kept by:

The General Council and Register of Osteopaths,
16 Buckingham Gate, London SW1
(Tel: 01–828 0601)

The following society has members who are graduates of the osteopathic and naturopathic schools listed above, and others who have trained at the École Européene d'Ostéopathie:

The Society of Osteopaths,
5 Guildford Road, Broadbridge Heath, Horsham,
West Sussex
(Tel: 0403–65087)

The members style themselves:

MSO   Member of the Society of Osteopaths

The school below was originally established to train French and Belgian psysiotherapists and practitioners unable to get such training in France, where there are restrictive laws on alternative medicine:

École Européene d'Ostéopathie,
104 Tonbridge Road, Maidstone, Kent
(Tel: 0622 671558)

Qualification
DO   Diploma in Osteopathy

Radionics, Radiesthesia (Medical Dowsing)

This association runs a two-year part-time-course, and keeps a register of members who have qualified:

The Radionic Association,
16A North Bar, Banbury, Oxon
(Tel: 0295–3183)

Qualifications
MRadA   Member of the Radionic Association
FRadA   Fellow of the Radionic Association

The following society restricts its membership to doctors and dentists with an interest in medical dowsing:

The Psionic Medical Society,
34 Beacon Hill Court, Hindhead, Surrey